F

Osteoporosis

How to Prevent
the Brittle-Bone Disease

by Wendy Smith
in consultation with Dr. Stanton H. Cohn

Produced by The Miller Press, Inc.

A Fireside Book
Published by Simon & Schuster, Inc.
New York

Published by Simon & Schuster, Inc.
Simon & Schuster Building
Rockefeller Center
1230 Avenue of the Americas
New York, New York 10020

FIRESIDE and colophon are registered trademarks
of Simon & Schuster, Inc.

Designed by Barbara Marks

Manufactured in the United States of America

Printed and bound by Fairfield Graphics

10 9 8 7 6 5 4 3 2 1

Library of Congress Cataloging in Publication Data

Smith, Wendy, date.
    Osteoporosis : how to prevent the brittle-bone disease.

    "A Fireside book."
    Bibliography: p.
    Includes index.
    1. Osteoporosis—Prevention. 2. Women—Diseases—
Prevention. 3. Self-care, Health. I. Cohn, Stanton H.
II. Title. [DNLM: 1. Osteoporosis—prevention & control—
popular works. WE 250 S6630]
RC931.O73S65   1985   616.7'1   85-1658

ISBN: 0-671-55252-X

Special thanks to Holly Reich of Hired Health, a private health and fitness consultancy based in New York City, for modeling services rendered.

Photographs by Ken Levinson

Acknowledgments

Many experts in the field of osteoporosis graciously consented to being interviewed for this book: I would like to extend my thanks to Dr. Louis V. Avioli, Dr. Bruce Ettinger, Dr. Robert P. Heaney, Dr. Michael Kleerekoper and Dr. B. Lawrence Riggs. Thanks also to Randi Aaron, who provided the menus and recipes in Chapter 4. My particular thanks to Angela Miller and David Gibbons of The Miller Press, whose hard work made it all happen.

Contents

Foreword

In recent years, the condition known as osteoporosis has received considerable public attention. Loss of bone with increasing age affects every person to a varying degree. Sex, race, genetic background, lifestyle, diet and physical activity are all factors in determining the strength of the bones of an individual. Women experience bone thinning at a rapid rate following menopause, and are more susceptible to fracture than men.

Bone is an active, living tissue. It is constantly remodeled by two forces, one which builds bone (formation) and the other which breaks it down (resorption). When the period of growth ends, the breakdown rate begins to exceed the building rate. Bone thinning occurs at a fairly slow rate prior to menopause. After menopause the rate of mineral loss increases, often with severe consequences. Inactivity and poor diets accelerate the loss of calcium and hasten the process.

At an April 1984 conference sponsored by the National Institute of Health, held in Washington, physicians and scientists came together to consider the best available approaches to the treatment and prevention of osteoporosis. The consensus arrived at by this group is discussed in this book.

Is the outlook all bleak? Not by any means. While there is no way at the present time by which demineralized bones can be restored to their former condition, research has shown that the loss can be slowed. Even more importantly, preventive measures can be taken early in one's life to lessen the effect of bone thinning. Good diet and physical exercise contribute to well-mineralized bones. We can help our children build a strong defense against osteoporosis, as well as help older persons withstand better the loss they have already sustained.

A word of caution is necessary. Moderation is the key to good health. If one has been very inactive, it is unwise to undertake a sudden intense program of exercise. There is no need to consume excessively large amounts of calcium, or to consume megadoses of vitamins. Four glasses of skim milk generally provide an adequate calcium intake without adding unnecessary fat. For those who cannot digest milk readily, other foods rich in calcium are available, and calcium supplements are also easily obtained. Exercise programs can be very simple. The best exercise is one that you enjoy. There is no need for special equipment—walking briskly is excellent for exercising the bones.

Particular attention to diet should be paid by adolescents. In the teen years and the early twenties, the desire to be thin or the single lifestyle which may favor fast foods can deprive the body of much needed calcium at a critical time. Similarly, diets of older persons may also be deficient because of loss of interest in producing well-balanced meals.

A number of therapeutic programs are being studied and are still under investigation. One such program with positive effects is estrogen replacement for postmenopausal women. The need for such treatment should be decided by an individual together with a physician, with consideration for the risks as well as the benefits.

Without doubt, the present interest in and understanding of osteoporosis will help the next generation maintain healthy bones in an easy, natural way.

DR. STANTON H. COHN
Senior Scientist and Head
Medical Physics Division
Medical Research Center
Brookhaven National Laboratory
and
Professor of Medicine
School of Medicine
Health Sciences Center
State University of New York
Stony Brook, New York

Preface

This book is the first one to outline clearly and simply what is known about osteoporosis, its prevention and its treatment in language the average person can understand. Osteoporosis has been intensively studied for a relatively short period, and there are still some areas of controversy regarding preventive measures and treatment. But there are also broad areas of agreement; more than enough information is available to help most women to radically reduce their chances of developing this potentially disabling disease. There may be research breakthroughs in the future, and arguments over details will continue, but these are the provenance of the experts, not the general public.

Naturally, if your efforts to prevent osteoporosis are going to involve drastic changes in your diet or lifestyle, you should consult your doctor to make sure these steps are wise—but I do mean *consult*. If there's one thing this book should tell you, it's that your health is in *your* hands. Ask for your doctor's opinion, consider it carefully, then make up your own mind. I hope this book will give you the facts you need to make an informed decision.

W.S.

PART I

What You Must Know About Osteoporosis

—

ONE

What Is Osteoporosis?

O steoporosis is a disease that accelerates the natural loss of bone mass accompanying aging, until the skeleton is so porous and fragile that a bone will break from the most minor trauma—lifting a heavy object, for example—or spontaneously fracture with no external trauma at all. It causes the unsightly and often painful "dowager's hump" seen on many elderly women: the spinal vertebrae become so weak that they collapse together in what is called a crush fracture, which can cause victims to become increasingly stooped and lose inches from their height. The wrist is another common site for osteoporosis-related breaks. Even more seriously, osteoporosis is the principal cause of hip fracture in the elderly; nearly 200,000 Americans over sixty-five fracture a hip annually, and 15–30 percent of them die from the ensuing complications.

A Major Public Health Problem

Experts estimate that 20 million people in the United States have osteoporosis, many without knowing it, and the disease is responsible for approximately 1.3 million fractures every year. A white woman who reaches the

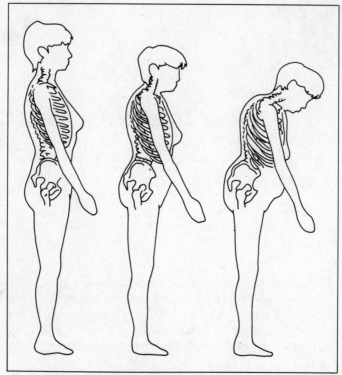

The progress of a crush fracture.

age of sixty has a 25–50 percent chance of sustaining at least one fracture before she dies (blacks are less susceptible). The complications arising from broken bones are the third leading cause of death in the population over sixty-five. Among those who live to be more than ninety, 32 percent of the women and 17 percent of the men will fracture a hip, and almost all of those injuries will be due to osteoporosis. The annual cost in terms of health care, social services and work hours lost has been calculated at $3.8 billion.

Clearly, osteoporosis is a serious public-health problem, and it's likely to get worse. The size of the population over forty-five is expected to increase by more than one third by the year 2000; if nothing is done to reduce the frequency of the disease, the number of osteoporosis-related fractures will rise to 1.7 billion by the end of the century. The costs associated with the disease will almost certainly increase in equal measure.

What Causes It?

The causes of osteoporosis aren't definitely known, although there are a couple of principal suspects. Given the complex nature of the disease and the varying responses to treatment, multiple causes are very likely, although none is yet unquestionably established. What *is* understood fairly exactly is the sequence of events leading to the drastic bone loss that accompanies osteoporosis.

Although it's natural to assume that something as hard and strong as bone is a solid, permanent substance, in fact it is a tissue that changes constantly. It's not even a single substance; there are two principal forms of bone. Trabecular bone is the spongy, metabolically active inner matrix that comprises about 20 percent of the total skeleton; the remaining 80 percent is cortical

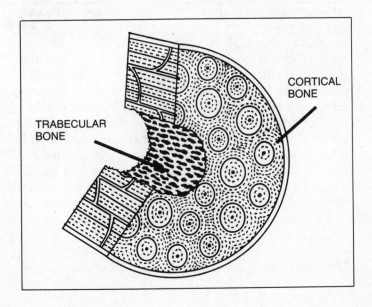

CORTICAL BONE

TRABECULAR BONE

(also called compact) bone—the thinner, smoother external envelope. Blood vessels and nerves flow through the bone tissue, which is impregnated with minerals, especially calcium and phosphorus. The proportions of the two types of bone vary greatly in different parts of the skeleton; their rates of age-related decline, susceptibility to fracture and response to treatment also differ widely.

Both types of bone are continually remodeling: removing minerals from the bone tissue and releasing them into the blood (resorption), taking minerals from the blood and building up new tissue (formation). These two activities are performed by two different cells: the osteoclasts make pits on the surface of the bones and remove a certain volume of it; the osteoblasts then refill the resorption cavities. This continual cycle of breaking down and building up bone is essential to the maintenance of a healthy skeleton.

Until age eighteen or so, bones grow because formation exceeds resorption. After that, although bones are no longer growing in size, the body is still adding to their density: 10–15 percent more material before the skeleton reaches its peak bone mass at approximately age thirty-five (even earlier for trabecular bone). A few years after this peak is reached, we begin to lose bone mass; as the osteoblasts become progressively less able to reconstitute resorbed bone, bone formation decreases. Loss of bone, therefore, is a normal part of the aging process; osteoporosis occurs when this bone loss is accelerated to abnormal levels and the critical level where osteoporosis begins is reached. "Osteoporosis is not a disease like tuberculosis that the patient either has or does not have," states one authority, "but corresponds to a dividing line chosen by the physician on a continuous scale." Often, the victim realizes she has osteoporosis only after she has broken a bone.

The Two Types of Osteoporosis
More and more often, doctors are dividing osteoporosis

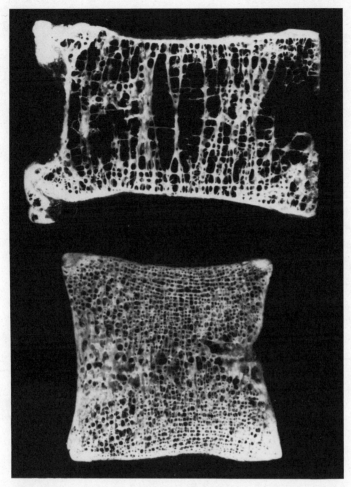

Osteoporotic bone (top) is much more porous than normal bone (bottom).

into two categories, both displaying the diminished bone mass that is the defining characteristic of the disease, but with different patterns of sex and age distribution and fracture location. Type I osteoporosis occurs six times as often in women, usually between the ages of fifty-five and seventy-five. Trabecular bone loss

23

is much greater than cortical, and the fractures usually occur in the spinal vertebrae (the classic crush fracture) or the wrist. Type II osteoporosis, which has "only" twice as many female as male victims, is a disease of older people, ages seventy to eighty-five. Trabecular and cortical bone are lost in equal amounts, and the most common fracture sites are the hips and other long bones; vertebral fractures occur with less frequency.

The distinction between the two kinds of osteoporosis is important, because evidence increasingly suggests that the two types have different primary causes and respond to different treatments. In order to understand these differences, it's necessary to know a bit more about the various minerals and hormones involved in bone remodeling.

The Role of Calcium and Hormones

One of the most vital elements in the remodeling process is the mineral calcium. During the years of peak adolescent growth, between 275 and 500 milligrams of calcium are deposited directly in the bones *each day*. After bone growth has ceased, but while bone density continues to develop, some 500 mg. of calcium daily are still required for skeletal maintenance.

Although 99 percent of the calcium in our bodies is stored in the skeleton, the remaining 1 percent circulating in the bloodstream is extremely important: it supports such essential nerve and muscle activities as heartbeat, blood clotting and muscle contraction. If the nerve cells aren't adequately bathed in calcium, muscle spasms can occur, creating a dangerous, potentially fatal situation. If you get enough calcium in your diet, both the bones and the blood are properly provided with this essential mineral. If you don't, the normal balance between bone formation and resorption will be disrupted: your body will withdraw calcium from the bones to circulate in the bloodstream, where it's more immediately important. The skeleton, in other words, serves as an enormous bank of calcium that assures the sufficiency of your blood calcium levels.

Three hormones are principally involved in the regulation of bone remodeling through their relationship with calcium. The parathyroid hormone (familiarly known as PTH) stimulates bone resorption; the peptide hormone calcitonin inhibits it. The secretion of both hormones is related to the level of calcium in the blood. When blood calcium is high, PTH secretions are low, because calcium levels are adequate and bone resorption doesn't need to be boosted to add calcium to the bloodstream. For the same reason, calcitonin secretions are high (inhibiting resorption) when calcium levels in the blood are high.

A drop in blood calcium levels will lead to an increase in PTH secretions, because more resorption is necesssary to supply the blood with calcium; it will also lead to a decline in calcitonin secretions, because resorption must not be repressed. The other effect of lower blood calcium levels is that the increased secretion of PTH facilitates the production of $1,25(OH)_2D_3$—more

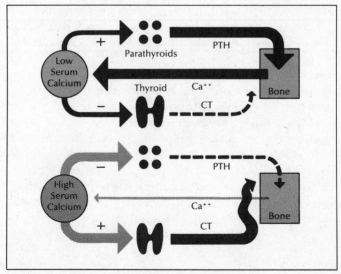

How calcium and hormones affect bone formation and resorption.

simply known as the hormonal form of vitamin D_3—which increases the efficiency of intestinal absorption of calcium to adapt to an insufficient dietary intake. In other words, while the PTH is stimulating the bones to release calcium into the bloodstream because of inadequate calcium levels there, it's also boosting the production of hormonal vitamin D_3, so that what little calcium is being ingested will be absorbed into the bones with maximum efficiency—thus minimizing the harmful effects of increased bone resorption.

One expert has called the effect of these three hormones (vitamin D must be converted to its hormonal form by the liver and kidneys in order to aid calcium absorption) on bone remodeling an "exquisite control system," and indeed it is. PTH and calcitonin secretions maintain circulating blood calcium at a constant level, no matter what the dietary intake of the mineral is, and hormonal vitamin D_3 does its best to get more calcium into your bones when resorption is increased. But below a certain level of calcium intake, vitamin D_3 can't help enough and there's a price to pay for the maintenance of a constant blood calcium level. The price is your bones.

Experts won't go so far as to label calcium deficiency the *cause* of osteoporosis, but a look at the mechanisms that regulate bone remodeling makes it clear that lack of dietary calcium triggers hormonal activity that encourages bone resorption. Animals placed on low-calcium but otherwise nutritionally complete diets have developed osteoporosis in experimental studies. The experiments haven't been reproduced with humans, for obvious ethical reasons, but the results with animals are suggestive. But calcium is only one element, albeit a very important one, in the complex interplay of factors involved in the accelerated bone loss that leads to osteoporosis. That brings us to the subject of which people are most likely to develop the disease.

TWO

Who Gets Osteoporosis?

Your Age

Old people, of course; osteoporosis is virtually exclusively a disease of aging. To begin with, it takes time for the effects of accelerated bone loss to be manifested in fractures, and osteoporosis basically has no symptoms other than broken bones. Certain physiological aspects of aging also increase the likelihood of osteoporosis. When you get older, you don't absorb calcium as efficiently as you did in your youth, and your diet tends to be calcium deficient as well, thereby enhancing the possibility of low blood calcium levels and increased bone resorption. Calcitonin secretions, which discourage resorption, decline with age, while PTH (parathyroid hormone) secretions, which stimulate resorption, have been found to increase with age in some (but not all) studies. With age you also need more vitamin D for the proper absorption of calcium, but you don't always get it, particularly if you are bedridden or institutionalized and aren't exposed often enough to the sun. (Vitamin-D formation is stimulated by sunlight on the skin.) Then, too, if you don't get enough exercise you are probably at greater risk of getting osteoporosis.

Your Sex

Women are far more susceptible than men to osteoporosis for a number of reasons. To begin with, their peak bone mass is 30 percent less than that of men; they simply have less bone to lose before they reach the critical, fracture-intensive level where osteoporosis is established. Although individual variations in age-related bone loss are great, in general women begin losing bone earlier than men and lose it faster. They have lower levels of calcitonin than men, too, so they don't inhibit bone loss as effectively.

Men lose bone at a constant rate of about .3 percent a year for cortical bone, slightly more for trabecular bone. Women, however, *begin* by losing about 1 percent of their trabecular and 1 percent of their cortical bone mass each year, and that rate accelerates dramatically after menopause. For three to seven years after menopause, bone loss averages 3 percent per year overall and can be as high as 8 percent in such areas as the lumbar vertebrae of the spine. These vertebrae are composed largely of trabecular bone, where accelerated bone loss occurs earlier and is greater than in cortical bone. Bone loss can reduce the female skeleton as much as 30 percent in the twenty years following menopause.

Women also have problems with calcium. They absorb it less efficiently than men, and their diet is almost always calcium-deficient. American women in general get well below the U.S. Recommended Dietary Allowance of 800 mg. a day, mostly because they avoid calcium-rich dairy products as too fattening. One expert estimates that teenage girls probably get less than half the RDA for adolescents of 1200 mg. daily and that adult women continue to underconsume calcium right up to menopause. Since calcium is an essential element in bone formation, these women enter menopause with a peak bone mass far below their genetic potential, making their age- and sex-accelerated bone loss even more devastating.

Another reason women are more prone to osteoporosis has to do with estrogen. Evidence suggests that estrogen protects the bone mass and even retards the rate of bone loss. At menopause, the amount of estrogen produced by most women drops dramatically, although there are wide individual variations in the extent of the drop. This sudden decline is almost certainly linked to the accelerated bone loss experienced by postmenopausal women; the fact that premenopausal removal of the ovaries, which manufacture estrogen, is often followed by osteoporosis also seems to support this relationship. Premenopausal women who are amenorrheic (not menstruating) are also at greater risk of osteoporosis, possibly due to reduced estrogen levels, and early menopause is considered a strong predictor for the development of osteoporosis.

Decline in estrogen levels has also been suggested as a factor in postmenopausal women's inefficient absorption of calcium. The idea is that lower estrogen levels stimulate the release of calcium from the bone, which decreases the secretions of PTH, which impairs the production of hormonal vitamin D_3 by the kidneys, which has a negative effect on calcium absorption. This theoretical chain of events has not been proven, but the reasoning is persuasive.

Family History

Women with a family history of osteoporosis are especially likely to develop the disease. Potential bone mass is a genetically determined factor; it sets an upper limit past which your bones won't grow. A family history of osteoporosis may indicate hereditary low bone mass, which means that age-related bone loss can lead quickly to osteoporosis.

Your Size

People with certain physical characteristics are at much greater risk of osteoporosis. Small stature, for example: short people have smaller skeletons and less bone mass, and less bone mass means greater peril from the natural bone loss that accompanies aging. Thin women are in greater danger than fat women; for some reason obesity guards against osteoporosis. There are several ideas about why being fat should make you less likely to develop this disease. One is that the extra weight actually stimulates formation of bone, because of the increased load the weight places on the skeleton. Reasonable stress on the skeleton is generally considered to be good for bone development. Another theory suggests that postmenopausal fat tissue has the ability to metabolize the body's weak androgens, a kind of hormone, into estrogen, which protects the bone mass.

Incidence Rates of Hip Fracture by Country or City and Sex

	Women	Men	Female/Male Ratio
United States (Rochester, Minn.)	101.6	50.5	2.01:1
New Zealand	96.8	35.2	1.79:1
Sweden	87.2	38.2	2.75:1
Jerusalem	69.9	42.8	1.63:1
United Kingdom	63.1	29.3	2.15:1
Holland	51.1	28.5	1.80:1
Finland	49.9	27.4	1.78:1
Yugoslavia*	39.2	37.9	1.03:1
Hong Kong	31.3	27.2	1.15:1
Yugoslavia+	17.3	18.2	0.95:1
Singapore	15.3	26.5	0.58:1
South African Bantu	5.3	5.6	0.94:1

*Low-calcium diet.
+High-calcium diet.

Ages are adjusted to United States population 1970. Source: Gallagher J. C., Melton L. M., Riggs B. L., and Bergstrath E. "Epidemiology of fractures of the proximal femur in Rochester, Minnesota," *Clin Orthop* 152: 35-43, 1980.

Your Skin Color

Women with fair skin are at much greater risk. Blacks are very seldom afflicted with osteoporosis, because they have greater bone mass than whites—10 percent greater on average, although there are wide individual variations. Among whites, fair-skinned people develop osteoporosis more often, but no one knows definitively why, although it is linked to the relationship between pigment and absorption of vitamin A.

Where You Live

Ironically, osteoporosis is a disease of privilege: you're more likely to develop it if you live in the affluent societies of North America, Europe or Scandinavia than if you inhabit the Third World. The Bantu tribe of South Africa, hardly the best fed or healthiest people in the world, had the lowest recorded incidence rates of hip fracture in a 1980 study that also looked at the populations of the United States, Sweden, Yugoslavia and Great Britain. No one really knows why the often ill-nourished peasants of the world's impoverished countries should be relatively free from osteoporosis while their better-fed sisters and brothers break bones left and right, but there are several possibilities. Many underdeveloped nations are largely nonwhite, and we've already learned that blacks are at less risk. Inhabitants of developed countries tend to live longer, and osteoporosis manifests its symptoms in old age (although it begins much earlier). The high protein intake and sedentary lifestyle of many people in industrial societies may also contribute to the higher incidence of osteoporosis.

Milk Allergy

Another group of people who stand a better chance of getting osteoporosis are the surprisingly large number of Americans who can't digest dairy products—or, more accurately, can't digest lactose, the milk sugar many of these products contain. Since they can't eat an entire food group that is the best dietary source of calcium, people with alactasia (so called because they're deficient in the enzyme lact*ase*, which breaks down lact*ose*) are at much greater risk of developing osteoporosis. Chapter 3 suggests a few simple ways to overcome this allergy.

Lack of Exercise

People who don't get any exercise are much more prone to osteoporosis. Studies of hospital patients with long-term illness have shown that immobilization and prolonged bed rest produce rapid bone loss. Conversely, regular weight-bearing exercise has been demonstrated in several studies to reduce bone loss and increase bone mass. (These studies are controversial, a point we'll come back to in Chapter 5.) Exercise may also increase the efficiency of calcium absorption. People who don't exercise have less muscle, and reduced muscle mass has been suggested as a factor contributing to osteoporosis.

What Is a Risk Factor?

None of the characteristics discussed above—age, sex, family history, size, weight, skin color, habitat, milk allergy, lack of exercise—is the *cause* of osteoporosis. The causes of the disease aren't yet known, although calcium deficiency and estrogen deficiency are the primary suspects. Being old, or female, or short, or thin, or fair, or sedentary is considered a *risk factor* for osteoporosis. That is to say, people with osteoporosis have been found to have these characteristics more often than they normally occur in the general population. This doesn't mean that if you're thin and fair you'll inevitably get osteoporosis—just that your chances are statistically somewhat greater.

There are many physical characteristics, lifestyle attributes and dietary habits that seem to increase the risk of osteoporosis, but it must be stressed that doctors by no means agree among themselves on how important the individual risk factors are. Some have been fairly definitely linked to osteoporosis through experimental studies; some rely more on anecdote or a physician's personal experience, neither of which is as convincing to other doctors as hard-and-fast evidence.

You Are What You Eat and Drink

DIETARY RISK FACTORS. The vast majority of risk factors, and those about which there are the most disagreements, are nutritional. There's no question that what you eat and drink can have a major effect on your bones, but often the exact mechanisms by which these substances affect the skeleton are unknown, or the data supporting their effect are sketchy.

ALCOHOL. One substance almost universally agreed to be a strong contributing factor to osteoporosis is alcohol, and there is some disturbing evidence that suggests you don't have to drink all that much. A recent study among men who drank socially—one or two drinks per day—found they had a twofold increased risk for osteoporosis. Alcohol both decreases the absorption of calcium and has a negative effect on the integrity of the bone.

NICOTINE. Cigarette smoking also carries with it an increased risk of osteoporosis, although the evidence is considered by some experts to be less convincing than that for alcohol. One recent study of women who smoked more than a pack a day showed they had less circulating estrogen, and estrogen deficiency is certainly a major factor in osteoporosis. Some doctors suggest that smoking cigarettes, like drinking alcohol, is simply bad for the bones: nicotine constricts blood vessels, and this may impair the nourishment of the bone.

CAFFEINE. Caffeine intake has also been linked to osteoporosis, mostly because it increases wastage of calcium. If you drink a lot of coffee, a higher proportion of calcium is excreted in your urine, which means that less is being absorbed into your bones. Aluminum-containing antacids have also been found to hamper calcium absorption.

These are the "bad-habit" risk factors; you don't *need* alcohol, cigarettes or caffeine (and certainly not aluminum), so if it's at all possible to give them up you'll be doing yourself and your bones a favor. There are a number of nutrients, however, that are essential to good health in the right quantities but if taken in excess can create an increased risk of osteoporosis.

PROTEIN. Probably the nutrient most generally accepted as a risk factor is protein, which increases urinary calcium. One expert estimates that a 130-pound woman needs to ingest only about 50 grams of protein a day: "any more is just sheer excess." The body takes any excess and stores most of it as fat, burning up the remaining nitrogen and sulphur and throwing them away—unfortunately, throwing away a lot of valuable calcium with them.

PHOSPHORUS. Phosphorus, which is generally present in foods that contain a lot of protein (such as beef, poultry and commercially baked breads), has been associated with protein as an osteoporosis risk, but this association is controversial. Many nutritionists state without qualification that too much phosphorus in the diet interferes with calcium absorption. Both minerals are present in a fixed ratio in bone, and the theory is that while bones absorb phosphorus well at high levels, the efficiency of calcium absorption declines at the same levels. Doctors are less convinced; studies have shown that phosphorus actually decreases urinary excretion of calcium, although it may enhance fecal loss. There's probably no need to be unduly concerned about phosphorus, but it's true that many American diets are higher than they need to be in this mineral, essential though it is. Certainly the substitution of diet soda (extremely high in phosphorus) for milk (high in calcium) is not a wise move.

OTHER DIETARY FACTORS. There are certain dietary factors about which the evidence is even less conclusive, often simply because there haven't been many relevant studies of the subject. What little we know about fat and osteoporosis, for example, suggests that small amounts of fat enhance calcium absorption, but large amounts impair it. Oxalic acid is another substance that has been reported to have an adverse effect on calcium absorption, which is a shame, since some of the foods containing it (spinach, parsley, beet greens) are also high in calcium. Some authorities believe that magnesium deficiency can result in abnormal bone formation, but a link between this and osteoporosis has not been established. If your diet is adequate in protein and calories, you are probably getting enough magnesium.

There are also a number of drugs that seem to cause bone loss and thus can lead to the development of osteoporosis. The ones most commonly used by older women, who are at most risk from osteoporosis, are probably corticosteroids. These drugs are frequently used to treat arthritis, so people who have that disease and are taking corticosteroids should be aware of the possible increased risk of osteoporosis.

The role of vitamin D in the genesis of osteoporosis is complex and will come up again in Chapters 3 and 4. The hormonal form of vitamin D_3 is very important for the proper absorption of calcium, and lack of vitamin D in the elderly may contribute to age-related bone loss. Very few normally active Americans, however, are deficient in vitamin D, thanks to fortified milk and our generally sunny climate.

How to Prevent It

Well, it all sounds pretty nebulous, doesn't it? The causes of osteoporosis aren't definitely known, and doctors don't agree on what physical characteristics and dietary substances put you at increased risk of developing the disease! How on earth can you protect yourself against something about which there are still so many questions?

The thing to remember is that medical researchers are, quite rightly, an extremely cautious group; they need a lot of evidence before they'll declare unequivocally that, for example, calcium deficiency causes osteoporosis. A woman who wants to lessen her chances of contracting the disease, however, doesn't have to be quite so stringent about the evidence. If a substance is suspected to contribute to the risk of osteoporosis, why not cut down on it? If the lack of a mineral or vitamin may make you more likely to contract the disease, why not try to make sure you get enough of it? (You should always be conscious of the dangers of recklessly increasing your consumption of any substance, however. Certain vitamins, including D, can build up to toxic levels in the blood very quickly.) Being aware of the risk factors for osteoporosis can help you avoid developing it.

To summarize, there are certain physical characteristics that seem to go hand in hand with osteoporosis:

Physical Risk Factors

Advancing age	Small stature
Female sex	Low body weight
Estrogen deficiency	Fair skin
Family history of osteoporosis	Alactasia (milk allergy)

You can't do much about those risk factors, of course, but there are some lifestyle and dietary factors that may also contribute to an increased risk of osteoporosis, and you *can* affect these by altering your habits and/or diet:

Lifestyle and Dietary Risk Factors

Calcium deficiency	High protein intake
Lack of exercise	High phosphorus intake
Excess alcohol consumption	High fat intake
Cigarette smoking	High oxalic-acid intake
Excess caffeine consumption	Magnesium deficiency
Consumption of aluminum-containing antacids	Use of corticosteroid drugs

Remember, not all of these risk factors are agreed upon by all doctors, and there is especial controversy over substances like phosphorus and magnesium.

It's a good idea to have these risk factors firmly in

mind, because there is *no cure* for osteoporosis. There are some treatments that retard the rate of bone loss, and a few experimental treatments may eventually be shown to actually restore some lost bone (see Chapter 8), but as yet there is no proven cure. The name of the game is prevention: building bigger and stronger bones now so you won't find yourself with a dangerously depleted skeleton later. How? That's the topic of the next section.

PART II

How to Prevent Osteoporosis

THREE

Building Peak Bone Mass
Before Menopause

The most important years in a woman's life for preventing osteoporosis are the decades *before* she
reaches age thirty-five, when peak bone mass is
achieved. Virtually all doctors agree that the single most
effective way to avoid developing osteoporosis is to
have the maximum possible bone mass at age thirty-
five. The more bone you have, the more you can afford
to lose in its inevitable age-related decline. Postmenopausal women can do many things to lower their rate of
bone loss (see Chapter 6), but it has yet to be proven
that anything you do after age thirty-five can give you
more bone. So, although osteoporosis is a disease of old
age, its prevention is in the hands of youth.

The two mainstays of osteoporosis prevention for
premenopausal women are a calcium-adequate diet and
weight-bearing exercise.

The Calcium-Adequate Diet
Although the U.S. Recommended Dietary Allowance
for adults is 800 mg. of calcium per day, a recent
National Health Institutes consensus development conference about osteoporosis suggested that 1000 mg. was

a more appropriate amount for premenopausal women; adolescents should get 1200 mg. a day. Chapter 1 explained how essential calcium is for building bone mass: as much as 500 mg. each day is deposited directly in the bones during peak adolescent bone growth, and the skeleton continues to require large amounts of calcium through the early adult years, when it's still adding bone density.

How Much Calcium?

	mg. per day
Teenagers	1200
Pregnant teenagers	1600
Women age twenty through menopause	1000
Pregnant women	1200
Postmenopausal women, no estrogen replacement therapy	1500
Postmenopausal women with estrogen replacement therapy	1000

Teenage Girls

Within the category of premenopausal women, there are two special groups that need even more calcium. The first, in chronological order, is teenage girls. Since their bones are still growing, they need more calcium than adults—1200 mg. a day, as noted above—and they also need to be discouraged from certain bad habits that strip their bodies of calcium and make it impossible for them to achieve their maximum peak bone mass. Women with adolescent daughters should try to discourage crash dieting in particular: drinking diet soda instead of milk is guaranteed to lower their calcium intake, and dieting in general tends to eliminate the "fattening" dairy products that are essential to a calcium-rich diet. Obviously, teenagers are also particularly susceptible to the forbidden glamour of alcohol and cigarettes, both of which are bad for the bones. Sensible mothers will undoubtedly be trying to convey the dangers of these tempting grown-up pastimes to their daughters in any case; the risk of osteoporosis is simply one more reason why your daughter shouldn't smoke or drink in excess.

Pregnant Women and Nursing Mothers

The second group of premenopausal women with an increased need for calcium is pregnant women and nursing mothers. During the last trimester of pregnancy, 200–300 mg. of calcium is deposited in the fetus each day. If the mother's dietary calcium isn't sufficient, her bones will give up calcium to ensure that the baby's needs are met. Similarly, if a nursing mother doesn't get enough calcium in her diet her bones will release the mineral in order to maintain a constant level of calcium in her milk. Mother Nature lends a hand to her fellow nurturers during this period: pregnant women absorb calcium more efficiently, getting more calcium from a glass of milk, for example, than they did before they were pregnant. All the same, calcium intake should be much higher during pregnancy. The USRDA for pregnant women and nursing mothers is 1200 mg. per day; pregnant teenagers, who need calcium for their own bone development as well as for their babies', should get 1600 mg. daily. The best possible source for calcium, as well as for the other nutrients you need during pregnancy and lactation, is milk—try to drink four glasses a day.

Risks of High Calcium Intake

The only risk associated with increased calcium intake in the premenopausal years is the possibility of kidney stones, a painful ailment of the urinary tract. Women with a family history of this problem should consult their doctor before boosting the calcium in their diet. For most people, however, doubling or even tripling a low calcium intake can only benefit their health, provided the calcium is absorbed properly. To be on the safe side, make sure you drink plenty of fluids.

*   *   *

Vitamin D, as we saw in Chapter 1, is essential for calcium absorption, but it's primarily older people who have problems with insufficient vitamin-D intake or improper metabolization. Chapter 6 deals with some of these special problems in detail.

Many of the risk factors discussed in Chapter 2, especially the ones associated with diet, increase your chances of developing osteoporosis because they increase the body's wastage of calcium. If you're really serious about getting enough calcium and absorbing it properly, then some of these elements should either be eliminated from your diet or at least be carefully monitored.

Alcohol, caffeine and nicotine are just plain bad for you and your bones; try to cut down on them. If you have an upset stomach, try drinking milk rather than taking aluminum-containing antacids. You need protein, of course, but there's no need to eat red meat at every meal; meat is high in protein, and excess protein leads to increased urinary excretion of calcium. High levels of phosphorus, fat and oxalic acid in your diet should probably be avoided. Keep an eye on your magnesium intake to make sure it's adequate (the RDA is 400 mg.); the effect of magnesium deficiency on osteoporosis is unproven, but magnesium is an essential mineral that's stored in your bones, and a connection is possible.

The best food sources for calcium, bar none, are dairy products. An eight-ounce glass of milk, skim or whole, has nearly 300 mg. of calcium, one ounce of cheddar cheese (a one-inch cube) has more than 200 mg., and one cup of yogurt has as much calcium as a glass of milk. Cottage cheese is also high in calcium, but it's also quite high in phosphorus. Swiss cheese has even more calcium than cheddar; in fact, basically all varieties of cheese are good sources of calcium. Ice cream and sour cream, fattening though they certainly are, are also high in calcium: eight ounces of ice cream has almost as much calcium as a cup of milk, and the same amount of sour cream has more. Puddings of all sorts have lots of calcium; custard and butterscotch are especially good.

Will I Gain Weight on a High-Calcium Diet?

Dairy products are higher in calories than some other foods—although skim milk is very low in calories—but the exercise you should be getting as the other mainstay of osteoporosis prevention ought to protect you against unwanted additional pounds. Frankly, exercise is always a better and healthier way to firm up and lose weight than are ridiculous diets you never stick with anyway. All the evidence indicates that no matter how much weight you lose on a crash diet, you'll put it all right back on as soon as you return to your normal eating habits. Permanent alteration of your diet combined with a regular program of exercise will help you achieve your desired weight—and it also happens to be the best method to ensure that you don't develop osteoporosis. Eliminating "fattening" dairy products isn't the healthiest way to stay thin.

What About Milk Allergies?

If you're one of those people who are milk-intolerant (one of the risk factors for osteoporosis discussed in Chapter 2), you should know that many drugstores sell lactase, the enzyme in which you're deficient. You can use it to treat milk so that you can comfortably digest its lactose. (Lactose is the milk sugar that unpleasantly affects the milk-intolerant; lactase is the enzyme that enables them to digest it.) Also, it's sometimes possible to buy low-lactose milk and cottage cheese. In some dairy products—yogurt, for example—the bacteria present have already digested the lactose, so you don't have to.

Calcium-Rich Foods

Other kinds of food are also high in calcium. Certain fish are excellent sources of calcium. A small serving of baked bass has 100 mg. of calcium; three and a half ounces of steamed scallops have 115 mg. Several types of canned fish are calcium-rich: herring, mackerel, red salmon, and sardines (provided you eat the soft bones too), and smelt. If you're fortunate enough to be attending a party where they're serving raw oysters as appetizers, have a half dozen or so; they'll give you nearly 100 mg. of calcium.

Nuts of all sorts have lots of calcium, although they're hardly the ideal source for calorie counters. For example, a mere ten unsalted almonds give you 25 mg. of calcium, along with 60 calories. Nuts aren't the perfect calcium source for a balanced diet, but the next time you're nibbling peanuts in a bar you can at least console yourself with the thought of all the calcium you're getting: roasted peanuts with their inner skin have 72 mg. of calcium in three and a half ounces.

Some vegetables are good sources of calcium, in particular the less commonly eaten leafy green vegetables. Try to develop a taste for collard greens, dandelion greens, turnip greens or kale. There are some more mundane vegetables with high calcium levels, provided they're eaten raw, such as celery, broccoli and spinach—but remember that oxalic-acid level in spinach and don't eat too much of it. I don't know how on earth anyone could eat a raw artichoke, but if you could you'd get 102 mg. of calcium from one large bud; it has only half that amount when cooked. Beans are also a decent source of calcium; most varieties, cooked or raw, will contain roughly 50 mg. of calcium in one cup.

Fruits aren't overall an especially good food group from which to get your calcium, but there are a few dried fruits that can give your intake a good boost (not to mention their salutary effect on your digestion)— namely dates, figs, prunes (uncooked) and raisins. Eat all the raisins you want; one cup has more than 100 mg. of calcium.

Tofu, a soybean product, is loaded with calcium in addition to all its other nutrients. Since the firm variety of this bean curd can be diced and stirred into all kinds of sauces and soups to add thickness, this is a particularly handy source of calcium. The soybeans from which tofu is made are a good, calcium-rich food as well.

Not all breads are a bountiful source of calcium, but certain kinds have substantial amounts—corn bread, for example. Buckwheat pancakes are also good. Some cereals provide calcium, although mothers would be better off eating their babies' cereal, which *really* has a lot. Oatmeal, Cream of Wheat and Post's Wheat Meal are all good, and of course if you add milk to these ready-to-eat brands they have even more calcium.

One exotic note: should you suddenly find a butcher shop that sells alligator meat on a regular basis, your calcium worries are over. One three-and-a-half-ounce piece contains 1231 mg. of calcium! Don't try nibbling on your handbag, though; the skin isn't where the calcium is.

Clearly, there are enough foods that supply large quantities of calcium so that you don't have to eat only dairy products in order to get enough in your diet. (Remember, however, that pregnant women should drink plenty of milk; it's the best source of many other minerals they need as well as calcium.) The time to develop a good diet is in the years before thirty-five, when what you eat contributes directly to building a better bone mass. Not only will you enter the postmenopausal danger years with more bone, you'll also have good eating habits that will continue to help keep your calcium level up as the process of age-related bone loss begins. There's no absolute proof that adequate calcium intake after menopause lowers the rate of bone loss—some doctors argue vehemently that it doesn't—but it certainly can't hurt. After menopause, when a woman's calcium requirement rises to 1500 mg. daily, it may be necessary to take calcium supplements in order to reach that level of intake. These supplements are discussed in detail starting on page 108. You can take calcium supplements before menopause if you need them. However, Dr. Robert P. Heaney of Creighton University insists that before menopause you should be able to get enough calcium from the food you eat: it's always better to get your nutrition from the grocery store rather than the drugstore.

FOUR

Calcium-Rich Menus and Recipes

———

Here are four weeks of sample menus, some calcium-rich recipes and some magical ways to add calcium to your diet that should help you get enough calcium without dying of diet boredom.

A Few Notes About the Menus

1. The measurements in general should be obvious; "1 cup" always means eight ounces.

2. You're going to have to drink one glass of milk almost every day in order to get enough calcium; milk is simply an essential food as far as getting enough vitamins and minerals is concerned. You certainly needn't worry about calories with skim milk, and if you don't like the taste—well, one glass goes down pretty quickly! If you're allergic, remember that lactase will help you digest the milk sugar in dairy products.

3. You'll notice that spinach appears frequently, even though it contains oxalic acid, which impairs calcium absorption. It's such a good source of calcium, though (and not that many vegetables are), that you should include it in your diet.

4. In general, the calorie counts of these meals are

very low. If you weigh 110 pounds, you should ingest between 1400 and 1850 calories a day—more if you're younger than thirty-five, less if you're older—to maintain your weight. All the daily menus contain less than 1850 calories, and only thirteen have more than 1400, which is the level of calories that women over fifty-five who weigh 110 should get daily.

5. I haven't included caffeine, which has a bad effect on calcium absorption, but I admit *I* couldn't get through the morning without my two cups of coffee! If you must indulge, try to keep your consumption down; coffee has virtually no calories, and no calcium, when it's drunk black. Decaffeinated coffee beans make a fairly decent cup of coffee these days. I recommend very little alcohol, because it too has a negative effect on calcium absorption, but if you drink your wine the way Europeans do at lunch, mixed with mineral water, you can enjoy a drink without quite as much bone-damaging alcohol. I understand that nonalcoholic beers taste more and more like the real thing as well. Remember, moderation is always a good idea.

Calcium and Calories

Food, serving size	Calcium, in mg.	Calories
Dairy		
Whole milk, 1 cup	298	180
Skim milk, 1 cup	300	90
Dry nonfat milk powder, 1 tbsp.	49	14
Nonfat fortified milk, 1 cup	359	105
Canned evaporated milk, ½ cup minus 1 tbsp.	252	137
Whole-milk yogurt, 1 cup	297	150
Low-fat yogurt, 1 cup	300	145
Buttermilk, 1 cup	285	99
Parmesan cheese, 1 oz.	320	110
Gruyère cheese, 1 oz.	287	115

Food, serving size	Calcium, in mg.	Calories
Edam cheese, 1 oz.	225	100
Swiss cheese, 1 oz.	272	95
American cheddar, 1 oz.	211	112
Part-skim Mozzarella, 1 oz.	207	80
Ricotta, part skim, 1 cup	669	340
Cottage cheese, regular	126	217
Cottage cheese, low fat	138	165
Cream cheese, 1 oz.	17	105
Other cheeses vary around 1 oz.	150–200	100–130
Light cream, ½ cup	180	350
Tofu, 3.5 oz.	128	80
Soybean milk	48	75

Soups (all servings are one cup)
Clam chowder

Manhattan	34	81
New England	91	130
Oyster stew	158	120
Cream of potato	62	115

Beans (all servings are one cup)

Soybeans, cooked	131	234
Yellow wax, cooked	63	280
Red kidney	70	218
White, cooked	95	224
Lima beans	55	262

Desserts

Blackstrap molasses, 1 tbsp.	137	43
Ice cream, 1 cup	176	300
Ice milk, 1 cup	176	184
Rice pudding with raisins, 1 cup	260	387
Eggnog, 1 cup	330	342
Tapioca pudding, 1 cup	173	221

Vegetables

Dandelion greens, 1 cup, raw	374	90
Collard greens, 1 cup	300	60

Food, serving size	Calcium, in mg.	Calories
Broccoli, 1 cup	144	40
Spinach, 1 cup	160	40
Green beans, 1 cup	62	30
Kale, 1 cup	206	43
Parsley, 1 cup, raw	122	26
Swiss chard, cooked, 1 cup	106	26
Okra, 1 cup	147	46
Pumpkin, cooked, 1 cup	60	61
Carrots, 1 cup	51	48
Sauerkraut, 1 cup	85	42
Alfalfa sprouts, 1 cup	51	41
Brussels sprouts, 1 cup	50	45
Onion, 1 cup	50	61
Cabbage, cooked, 1 cup	64	29
Beet, turnip, mustard greens; chicory, escarole, carrot, celery tops, 1 cup	100–200	25
Turnips, 1 cup	34	36

Fruits

Orange, one	54	64
Watermelon, 4" x 8" slice	65	156
Dried dates, 10 pitted	60	274
Dried apricots, 1 cup	100	338
Rhubarb, 1 cup	20	117
Raisins, 1 cup	102	477
Strawberries, 1 cup	32	56

Teas (per 100 g.)

Bancha, all good sources	720	—
Black	460	—
Green	440	—

Seaweeds (per 100 g.)

Miso	140	*
Agar-agar	400	*
Dulse	1,170	*
Hijiki	1,400	*
Kelp	1,093	*

Food, serving size	Calcium, in mg.	Calories
Kombu	800	*
Nori	260	*
Wakame	1,300	*
*Not available.		
Fish		
Sardines, 1/4 lb.	496	232
Salmon, canned, 1 cup	431	310
Salmon, fresh, 1/4 lb.	90	246
Mackerel, canned, 1 cup	338	384
Herring, canned, 1 cup	65	416
Herring, fresh, 1/4 lb.	294	200
Oysters, canned, 1 cup	57	158
Oysters, fresh, 1/4 lb.	106	75
Snails, 35 oz.	170	90
Haddock, 4 oz.	45	180
Most other fish, 4 oz.	25–50	180
Nuts and Seeds		
Hazelnuts, 1/2 cup	141	428
Brazil nuts, 1/2 cup	180	458
Almonds, 1/2 cup	166	425
Walnuts, 1/2 cup	50	325
Sesame seeds, 1/2 cup	83	437
Sunflower seeds, 1/2 cup	87	406

Four Weeks of Calcium-Rich Menus

Week One

Monday

BREAKFAST

Cooked oatmeal, 1 cup, with	53	130
Skim milk, 4 oz.	150	45
Grapefruit juice, 8 oz.	22	98

LUNCH

Plain low-fat yogurt, 8 oz.	300	145

Week One	Calcium, in mg.	Calories
DINNER		
Steamed scallops, 3½ oz.	115	112
Steamed broccoli, three 5½" stalks	309	96
Scalloped potatoes, ½ cup	66	127
Skim milk, 8 oz.	300	88
Totals	1315	841

Tuesday
BREAKFAST		
Corn muffin, 1 large, with	100	260
Butter, 2 tbsps.	8	216
Orange juice, 8 oz.	27	111
LUNCH		
Salad:		
Raw spinach, 3½ oz.	93	26
Cubed Swiss cheese, 2 oz.	518	208
Raw green beans, ½ cup	28	16
Tomato, ½	7	11
Raw peas, ¼ cup	9	28
DINNER		
Spaghetti, 1 cup, with	16	216
Tomato sauce, ½ cup	10	45
Grated Parmesan cheese, ½ oz.	160	55
Cooked kale, 1 cup	206	45
Cooked okra, 1 cup	146	46
Totals	1328	1283

Wednesday
BREAKFAST		
Cooked Cream of Wheat, 1 cup, with	13	130
Skim milk, 4 oz.	150	45
Apple juice, 8 oz.	15	116

Week One	Calcium, in mg.	Calories

LUNCH

	Calcium, in mg.	Calories
Canned salmon (with bones), 3 oz., with	372	174
Lemon juice, 1 tbsp.	1	4
Swiss cheese, 1 oz., on	272	95
Italian bread, toasted, 2 slices	6	110
Skim milk, 8 oz.	300	90

DINNER

Chicken stir-fried with vegetables:

	Calcium, in mg.	Calories
Chicken breast, 4 oz.	10	120
Broccoli, one 5½" stalk	103	32
Cubed tofu, 2 oz.	72	40
Celery, 1 outer stalk	25	9
Green beans, ½ cup	31	16
Carrot, ½	18	21
Rice, ½ cup	8	82
Oyster sauce to taste	*	*
Totals	1396	1084

*The nutritional contents of oyster sauce weren't listed in any of the standard volumes of food values; I guess oyster sauce doesn't qualify as a "commonly used" item. In any case, the calcium content is probably pretty high, because oysters are rich in calcium, but the calorie count is undoubtedly hefty as well.

Thursday

BREAKFAST

	Calcium, in mg.	Calories
English muffin, 1 (2 halves), with	0	138
Melted Cheddar cheese, 1½ oz.	316	168
Grape juice, 8 oz.	28	165

LUNCH

	Calcium, in mg.	Calories
New England clam chowder, 2 cups	180	260

DINNER

	Calcium, in mg.	Calories
Baked macaroni and cheese, 1 cup	407	506
Cooked artichoke, 1, with	51	44
Melted butter, 2 tbsps.	8	216
Lemon juice, 1 tbsp.	1	4

Week One	Calcium, in mg.	Calories
Skim milk, 8 oz.	300	90
Totals	1291	1591

Friday
BREAKFAST

	Calcium, in mg.	Calories
Wheat flakes, 1 cup, with	12	106
Skim milk, 4 oz.	150	45
Pineapple-grapefruit juice, 8 oz.	13	123

LUNCH
Grilled cheese sandwich:

	Calcium, in mg.	Calories
American cheese, 1½ slices (1 oz.)	195	107
Whole-wheat bread, 2 slices	44	140

DINNER

	Calcium, in mg.	Calories
Broiled oysters, 1 doz.	188	168
Rice, ½ cup	8	82
Salad:		
Raw spinach, 3½ oz.	93	26
Raw broccoli, one 5½" stalk	103	32
Raw yellow beans, ½ cup	28	14
Alfalfa sprouts, 1 oz.	12	10
Cucumber, ½ (unpared)	13	8
Cubed Swiss cheese, 1 oz.	272	105
Skim milk, 8 oz.	300	90
Totals	1431	1050

Saturday
BREAKFAST

	Calcium, in mg.	Calories
Corn Bread,* two 2" squares	174	200
Tomato juice, 8 oz.	17	45

LUNCH

	Calcium, in mg.	Calories
Canned sardines (with bones), ¼ lb. on	496	232
Toasted rye bread, 2 slices	34	140

*See page 73.

Week One	Calcium, in mg.	Calories
Skim milk, 8 oz.	300	90
DINNER		
Beef Stroganoff:		
Stew beef, ½ lb.	15	294
Stroganoff sauce with ½ cup sour cream	122	454
Enriched noodles, 1 cup	16	200
Cooked collard greens, 1 cup	304	60
Totals	1490	1715

Sunday

BREAKFAST

Buckwheat pancakes, 4" diameter, 2 with	118	120
Butter, 2 tbsps.	8	216
Maple syrup, 3 tbsps.	62	150
Orange, 1	54	64

LUNCH
Salad:

Raw turnip greens, ½ cup	123	14
Celery, 1 cup, diced	47	20
Cubed tofu, 2 oz.	72	40
Broccoli, one 5½" stalk	103	32
Carrot, ½	18	21
Cubed Edam cheese, 1 oz.	225	105

DINNER

Broiled loin pork chop, 4 oz. (cut the fat off)	9	267
Cooked zucchini, 1 cup	45	25
Lima beans, ½ cup	26	131
Skim milk, 8 oz.	300	90
Dried figs, 5, for dessert	126	275
Totals	1336	1570

	Calcium, in mg.	Calories
Week Two		
Monday		
BREAKFAST		
Corn muffin, 1 small	50	130
Orange, 1	54	64
Skim milk, 8 oz.	300	90
LUNCH		
Swiss-cheese sandwich:		
Swiss cheese, 2 oz.	540	200
Lettuce and 1 tomato slice	20	10
Whole-wheat bread, 2 slices	45	140
Apple, 1	12	90
Brazil nuts, 1/4 cup	90	214
DINNER		
Vegetarian soup, 1 cup	20	80
Baked chicken, 4 oz.	10	120
Sautéed collard greens, 1 cup	300	180
Lima beans, 1/2 cup	27	130
Whole-wheat roll, 1	20	100
Totals	1488	1548
Tuesday		
BREAKFAST		
Cooked oatmeal, 1 cup, with	53	130
Skim milk, 4 oz.	150	45
Dried apricots, 1/4 cup	30	85
Cinnamon, 1 tsp.	—	—
Grapefruit, 1/2 cup	16	43
LUNCH		
Pizza, 1 small slice	150	250
Apple, 1	12	90
DINNER		
Stuffed Tomato*	305	192
Steamed spinach, 1 cup	160	40
Steamed broccoli, 1 cup	144	40

*See page 76.

Week Two	*Calcium, in mg.*	*Calories*
Whole-wheat roll, 1	20	90
SNACK		
Skim milk, 8 oz.	300	90
Oatmeal raisin cookies, 2	6	126
Totals	1346	1223

Wednesday

BREAKFAST

Shredded wheat, 1 loaf	11	90
Skim milk, 8 oz.	300	90
Banana, ½	6	63

LUNCH

Grilled Swiss-cheese sandwich:		
Swiss cheese, 2 oz.	544	110
Whole-wheat bread, 2 slices	45	140
Tomato, 3 slices	5	8
Salad:		
Romaine lettuce, 1 cup	30	10
Tomato, 1 small	20	33
Cucumber, ¼	13	8
Alfalfa sprouts, ½ cup	25	20
Italian dressing, 1 tbsp.	2	90

DINNER

Broiled salmon steak, 4 oz., with garlic	90	310
Oil, 1 tbsp. for broiling	—	125
Steamed broccoli, 1 cup	144	40
Brussels sprouts, 1 cup	50	45
Brown rice, 1 cup	18	178
Totals	1303	1360

Thursday

BREAKFAST

Energy Shake*	250	170

*See page 73.

Week Two	Calcium, in mg.	Calories
LUNCH		
Sardine plate:		
Sardines, 4 oz.	496	232
Romaine lettuce	15	5
Tomato	20	33
Carrot sticks	25	25
Onion slices	13	15
Black bread, 1 slice	27	90
Oil and vinegar, 2 tbsps.	2	125
DINNER		
Steamed vegetables:		
Broccoli, 1/2/ cup	72	20
Kale, 1/2 cup	103	22
Collard greens, 1/2 cup	150	30
Carrot, 1/2 cup	25	25
Tofu, 4 oz.	144	90
over Brown rice, 1 cup	18	178
top with		
Melted Jarlsberg cheese, 1 oz.	250	90
SNACK		
10 pitted dates	60	274
Totals	1670	1424
Friday		
BREAKFAST		
Grape Nuts cereal, 1 oz.	—	100
Skim milk, 8 oz.	300	90
Strawberries, 1/2 cup	15	26
Orange juice, 8 oz.	27	112
LUNCH		
Plain low-fat yogurt, 8 oz.	300	145
Banana, 1	12	120
Bran muffin, 1	80	200
DINNER		
Salmon Broccoli Loaf*, 4 oz.	334	225

*See page 75.

Week Two	Calcium, in mg.	Calories
Sweet potato, 1 small	46	160
Salad:		
Leaf lettuce, Boston	30	10
Tomato, 1 small	20	33
Alfalfa sprouts, 1 cup	50	40
Carrots, ½ cup	25	25
Brown Rice Pudding*, 1 cup	139	126
Totals	1378	1412

Saturday

BREAKFAST

Scrambled egg, 1, with	27	82
Lowfat cottage cheese, ¼ cup	35	45
Grapefruit juice, 4 oz.	11	50
Skim milk, 8 oz.	300	90

LUNCH

New England clam chowder, 1 cup	91	130
Oyster crackers	2	33

DINNER

White wine, 1 glass	—	100
Oysters on half shell, 6	106	75
Broiled salmon steak, 4 oz.	90	246
Steamed spinach, 1 cup	160	40
Steamed broccoli, 1 cup	144	40
Baked potato, 1	14	90
Yogurt and chives, 2 tbsps.	50	25
Ice milk, 1 cup	176	180
Totals	1228	1296

Sunday

BREAKFAST

French Toast†, topped with	142	225
Maple syrup, 3 tbsps.	62	150
Skim milk, 8 oz.	300	90

*See page 72.
†See page 74.

Week Two	Calcium, in mg.	Calories
LUNCH		
Vanilla yogurt, 8 oz.	300	200
Apple, 1	12	90
DINNER		
Shrimp stir fried with vegetables:		
Fresh shrimp, 4 oz.	72	100
Broccoli, one 5½" stalk	103	32
Celery, 1 stalk	25	9
Kale, 1 cup	206	40
Green beans, ½ cup	30	15
Brown rice, ½ cup	9	90
Sesame oil, 1 tbsp.	—	125
Soy sauce to taste	*	*
Total	1261	1166

*Not available.

Week Three

Monday
BREAKFAST

	Calcium, in mg.	Calories
Whole-wheat bread, 1 slice	22	70
Cream cheese, 1 oz.	17	105
Orange, 1	54	64
LUNCH		
Vegetable salad:		
Spinach, 1 cup	150	40
Mushrooms, ¼ cup	1	5
Alfalfa sprouts, ½ cup	25	20
Broccoli, ½ cup	72	20
Onion, ¼ cup	15	13
Tofu, cubed, 2 oz.	73	45
Swiss cheese, 1 oz.	272	100
Chickpeas, ¼ cup	33	60
Tofu Dressing[†], 2 oz.	50	30

†See page 78.

Week Three	Calcium, in mg.	Calories
Skim milk, 8 oz.	300	90
DINNER		
Tomato juice, 8 oz.	17	46
Broiled haddock, 4 oz.	45	180
Steamed green beans, 1 cup	62	30
Baked potato, with	14	90
Yogurt and chives, 2 tbsps.	50	25
Totals	1272	1033

Tuesday

BREAKFAST		
Poached egg	27	82
Whole-wheat toast, 1 slice	22	70
Skim milk, 8 oz.	300	90
LUNCH		
Manhattan clam chowder, 8 oz.	34	81
Tuna salad sandwich:		
Tuna fish, ½ cup	15	125
Mayonnaise, 2 tsps.	1	75
Whole-wheat bread, 2 slices	44	140
Lettuce, tomato	10	10
DINNER		
Quick Pasta Primavera*	697	503
Lettuce, 1 cup	10	15
Tomato, 1 medium	20	33
Onion, ¼ cup	12	20
Italian dressing, 2 tsps.	4	166
Totals	1196	1410

*See page 74.

Wednesday

BREAKFAST		
Bran muffin, 1	80	200
Orange, 1	54	64
Skim milk, 8 oz.	300	90

Week Three	Calcium, in mg.	Calories
LUNCH		
Salmon sandwich:		
Canned salmon, ½ cup	215	155
Mayonnaise, 2 tsps.	1	75
Lettuce, tomato	10	10
Cheddar cheese, 1 oz.	204	114
Rye bread, 2 slices,	34	160
Apple, 1	12	90
DINNER		
Spinach Squares*	169	82
Spaghetti, ½ cup	6	80
Tomato sauce, ½ cup	8	50
Grated Parmesan cheese, 3 tbsps.	207	69
Salad:		
Lettuce, 1 cup	30	10
Tomato, 1 medium	20	33
Cucumber, ½ cup	8	13
Tofu Dressing+, 2 oz.	50	30
Totals	1408	1325

*See page 75.
+See page 78.

Thursday
BREAKFAST

Cornflakes, 1 cup	2	97
Banana, ½	6	63
Skim milk, 8 oz.	300	90

LUNCH

Cantaloupe, ½	24	80
Low-fat cottage cheese, ½ cup	70	90
Whole-wheat AK-MaK Crackers, 4	21	117

DINNER
Chicken Parmesan:

Chicken breast, 4 oz.	10	120
Egg, 1	27	80

Week Three	Calcium, in mg.	Calories
Oil, 1 tbsp.	—	125
Tomato sauce, ½ cup	8	50
Mozzarella cheese, 2 oz.	414	160
Sautéed Swiss chard, 1 cup	106	26
Oil, 1 tbsp. (for sautéing)	—	125
Spaghetti, ½ cup	6	80
Tomato sauce, ½ cup	8	50
Grated Parmesan cheese, 1 tbsp.	69	23
Ice milk, 1 cup	176	180
Totals	1247	1535

Friday

BREAKFAST

Poached egg	27	82
Whole-wheat bread, 1 slice	22	70
Skim milk, 8 oz.	300	90

LUNCH

Pita sandwich:

Pita bread, 1 piece	40	140
Canned salmon, ½ cup	215	155
Grated cheese, 1 oz.	207	100
Spinach, ½ cup	80	20
Alfalfa sprouts, ½ cup	25	20
Grated carrot, ½ cup	25	25
Tofu Dressing*, 2 oz.	50	30
Orange, 1	54	64

DINNER

Oyster stew	158	120
Broiled scallops, 4 oz.	30	100
Okra, 1 cup	146	46
Baked potato, 1	14	90
Parmesan cheese, 3 tbsps.	207	69
Totals	1600	1221

*See page 78.

Week Three	Calcium, in mg.	Calories
Saturday		
BREAKFAST		
Buckwheat pancakes, 2, with	198	180
Maple syrup, 3 tbsps.	62	150
Grapefruit, ½	16	41
Skim milk, 8 oz.	300	90
LUNCH		
Apple, 1	12	90
Jarlsberg cheese, 2 oz.	500	180
Rice cakes, 2	—	75
DINNER		
Swordfish, broiled, 4 oz.	22	150
Green beans, 1 cup	62	30
Broccoli, 1 cup	144	40
Scalloped potato au gratin with 1		
cup cheese	311	355
Totals	1627	1381
Sunday		
BREAKFAST		
Omelet:		
Egg, 1	27	82
Egg white, 1	3	17
Swiss cheese, 1 oz.	272	95
Spinach, ½ cup	80	20
Whole-wheat roll, 1	22	90
Skim milk, 8 oz.	300	90
LUNCH		
Fruit cup, 1 cup	50	64
Yogurt	300	145
DINNER		
Tomato soup, 1 cup	67	69
Spaghetti, 1 cup	12	180
Tomato sauce, ½ cup	8	50
Steamed broccoli, 1 cup	144	40

	Calcium, in mg.	Calories
Week Three		
Steamed zucchini, 1 cup	45	25
Grated Parmesan cheese, 3 tbsps.	207	69
Totals	1537	1036

Week Four

Monday
BREAKFAST

	Calcium, in mg.	Calories
Low-fat yogurt, 1 cup, mixed with	300	145
Banana, ½	6	63
Granola, ¼ cup	5	98

LUNCH

	Calcium, in mg.	Calories
Broiled hamburger, 4 oz., with	13.5	304
Cheese, 1 oz.	195	103
Romaine lettuce, 1 cup	15	10
Tomato, 1	20	33
Cabbage, ½ cup	17	10
Oil and vinegar, 1 tbsp.	—	60
Enriched bun, 1	30	120
Skim milk, 8 oz.	300	90

DINNER

	Calcium, in mg.	Calories
Walnut Cheese Loaf*, 1 slice	116	230
Steamed collard greens, 1 cup, topped with	300	60
Sesame seeds, 1 tbsp.	13	72
Whole-grain bread, 1 slice	20	80
Applesauce, ½ cup	5	50
Totals	1355	1528

*See page 79.

Tuesday
BREAKFAST

	Calcium, in mg.	Calories
Shredded wheat, 1 average loaf	37	90
Skim milk, 4 oz.	150	45
Raisins, ¼ cup	25	120
Orange juice, 4 oz.	14	66

Week Four	Calcium, in mg.	Calories
LUNCH		
French onion soup with cheese, 1 bowl	218	162
Salad:		
Romaine lettuce, 1 cup	15	10
Zucchini, ½ cup	18	13
Watercress, ½ cup	35	25
Dressing:		
Vinegar, 2 tbsps.	2	4
Lemon juice, fresh, 2 tbsps.	—	10
Grated Parmesan cheese, 1 tbsp.	69	23
DINNER		
Stuffed Tomato with Salmon*	504	332
Steamed Brussels sprouts, 1 cup	50	45
Whole-wheat roll (small), 1	37	90
Totals	1174	1035

*See page 77.

Wednesday

	Calcium, in mg.	Calories
BREAKFAST		
Corn Bread†, one 2″ × 2″ piece	87	101
Low-fat cottage cheese, ½ cup	69	90
Grapefruit, ½	16	45
LUNCH		
Sardine Salad‡	510	246
Whole-wheat bread, 1 slice	22	70
Mustard to taste	—	—
Lettuce	5	5
Tomato	10	10
Skim milk, 8 oz.	300	90
Apple, 1	12	90
DINNER		
Tomato soup made with milk, 1 cup	67	72

†See page 73.
‡See page 75.

Week Four	Calcium, in mg.	Calories
Brown rice, ¹/2 cup	9	90
Soybeans, ¹/2 cup	65	117
Cooked cabbage, 1 cup	64	29
Kale, 1 cup sautéed in Oil, 1 tsp.	206	43
Top with Grated Cheddar cheese, 1 oz.	204	114
Totals	1646	1212

Thursday

BREAKFAST

Energy Shake*	174	150
Bran muffin, 1 small	80	200

LUNCH

Spinach Salad:

Raw spinach, 2 cups	320	80
Raw mushrooms, ¹/2 cup	2	10
Hard-boiled egg, 1	27	82
Swiss cheese, 1 oz.	272	95
Tomato, 1	10	33
Alfalfa sprouts, ¹/2 cup	25	23
Low-calorie bleu-cheese dressing, 2 tbsps.	20	30
Whole-wheat bread, 1 slice	22	80

DINNER

Veal Parmesan+	223	468
Spaghetti, ¹/2 cup	6	90
Tomato sauce, ¹/2 cup	8	50
Grated Parmesan cheese, 1 tbsp.	69	23
Steamed kale, 1 cup	206	43
Italian bread, 1 slice	9	60
Totals	1473	1517

*See page 73.
+See page 78.

Week Four	Calcium, in mg.	Calories
Friday		
BREAKFAST		
Wheat Meal cereal, 1 cup	17	110
Skim milk, 8 oz.	300	90
Dates, 5	30	137
Orange, 1	54	64
LUNCH		
Chicken salad, ½ cup	20	280
Rye bread, 2 slices	34	140
Lettuce (on sandwich)	10	10
Alfalfa sprouts	10	10
DINNER		
Oysters, 1 doz.	212	150
Broiled haddock, 4 oz., cooked with lemon and	45	100
Oil, 1 tbsp.	—	125
Baked potato with	14	90
Parmesan cheese, 2 tbsps.	140	46
Steamed green beans, 1 cup	62	30
SNACK		
Apple, 1	12	90
Skim milk, 8 oz.	300	90
Totals	1250	1552
Saturday		
BREAKFAST		
Waffle, 1 (5½" diameter)	85	209
Low-fat yogurt, ½ cup	150	72
Banana, ½	6	63
Maple syrup, 1 tbsp.	33	50
Orange juice, 4 oz.	14	56
LUNCH		
Skim milk, 8 oz.	300	90

Week Four	*Calcium, in mg.*	*Calories*
Low-fat Cottage Cheese Dip*, 2 oz.		
with	48	45
Raw broccoli, 1 cup	144	40
Raw cauliflower, ½ cup	13	15
Raw zucchini, 1 cup	36	25
Rice cakes, 2	—	75
DINNER		
New England clam chowder, 1 cup	91	130
Poached salmon, 4 oz.	90	246
Sautéed Swiss chard, 1 cup	106	26
Sautéed carrots, 1 cup	51	48
Oil, 1 tbsp.	—	125
Whole-wheat bread, 1 slice	22	70
Strawberries, 1 cup	32	56
Totals	1221	1441

Sunday

BREAKFAST

	Calcium, in mg.	Calories
Asparagus cheese omelet (made in nonstick pan):		
Eggs, 2	54	164
Cheddar cheese, 1 oz.	211	112
Cut-up asparagus spears, 4	21	20
Pumpernickel bread, 2 slices	54	160
Cream cheese, 1 oz.	17	105

LUNCH

Miso Soup⁺	223	80
Rice cakes, 2	—	75

DINNER

Stir-fried chicken broccoli:		
Cubed chicken, 4 oz.	10	120
Broccoli, three 5½" stalks	309	66
Sesame oil, 2 tbsps.	—	125
Soy sauce, 2 tbsps.	30	24

*See page 73.
⁺See page 74.

Week Four	Calcium, in mg.	Calories
Brown rice, ½ cup	9	90
Orange, 1	54	64
SNACK		
Skim milk, 8 oz.	300	90
Oatmeal raisin cookies, 2	10	130
Totals	1302	1425

Calcium-Rich Recipes

BROWN RICE PUDDING	Calcium, in mg.	Calories
Cooked brown rice, 2 cups	36	360
Skim milk, 1 cup	300	90
Whole egg, 1	27	82
Egg white, 1	3	17
Vanilla, 1 tsp.	—	—
Raisins, ½ cup	50	232
Blackstrap molasses, 3 tbsps.	311	130
Honey, 1 tbsp.	1	64
Chopped walnuts, ¼ cup	25	162
Lemon peel, 1 tbsp.	1	—
Low-fat yogurt, 1 cup	300	145
Cinnamon, 1 tsp.	28	6
Allspice, ½ tsp.	6	3
Dash of nutmeg	—	—
Chopped apple, 1 cup	12	90
Eight servings:	1108	1106
One serving:	139	124

Combine eggs, milk, honey, molasses and vanilla in blender. Put into a large bowl. Stir in the rice. Add remaining ingredients, except the yogurt. Mix well. Pour into 8-inch pan which has been lightly brushed with oil. Bake at 250° for 25 minutes. Stir every 10 minutes while baking. Cool 15 minutes and stir in yogurt. Add more cinnamon or allspice to taste. Serve hot or cold.

Corn Bread

	Calcium, in mg.	Calories
Corn meal, 1 cup	20	427
Whole-wheat flour, 1 cup	41	333
Baking powder, 2 tbsps.	—	—
Egg, 1	27	82
Molasses, ¼ cup	411	130
Corn oil, 3 tbsps.	—	375
Skim milk, 3 cups	300	90
Total	900	270
One 2" × 2" piece:	87	100

Combine dry ingredients, then wet ingredients. Mix together. (Mixture will be very watery.) Pour into greased 9" × 9" pan. Bake at 350° for 50 minutes.

Cottage Cheese Dip

	Calcium, in mg.	Calories
Low-fat cottage cheese, 8 oz.	138	165
Low-fat yogurt, 2 oz.	75	37
Lemon juice, 2 tbsps.	2	8
Chives, ½ tsp.	—	—
Dill, ½ tsp.	16	3
Dijon mustard, ½ tsp.	—	8
Basil, ¼ tsp.	8	2
Total	239	223
One 2-oz. serving:	48	45

Energy Shake

	Calcium, in mg.	Calories
Skim milk, 4 oz.	150	45
Low-fat yogurt, 2 oz.	75	36
Banana, ½	6	60
Strawberries, ½ cup	19	25
Vanilla, 1 tsp.	—	—
Bran, 1 tsp.	—	4
Ice cubes	—	—
One serving:	174	150

Mix together in blender.

French Toast

	Calcium, in mg.	Calories
Egg, 1 small	22	65
Skim milk, 1/4 cup	75	20
Vanilla, 1/4 tsp.	—	—
Whole-wheat bread, 2 slices	45	140
Cinnamon	—	—
Total	142	225

Beat egg and milk; add vanilla. Dip bread into batter. Cook on hot nonstick pan until brown on one side, turn, brown on the other side. Sprinkle with cinnamon.

Miso Soup

	Calcium, in mg.	Calories
Water, 12 oz.	—	—
Miso paste, 1 tbsp.	14	25
Cubed tofu, 2 oz.	73	45
Seaweed wakame, 1 oz.	130	20
Total	217	80

Soak seaweed in plain water. Set aside for 5 minutes. Boil the water, add the miso paste, tofu and seaweed. Heat and serve.

Quick Pasta Primavera

	Calcium, in mg.	Calories
Pasta, 2 oz.	10	210
Kale, 1 cup	206	43
Broccoli, 1 cup	144	40
Tomato sauce, 1 cup	17	100
Grated Parmesan cheese, 1 oz.	320	110
Two servings:	697	503

Cook pasta. Steam vegetables. Mix pasta and vegetables together. Top with sauce and cheese. Serves two.

SALMON BROCCOLI LOAF

	Calcium, in mg.	Calories
Canned salmon, 2 cups	862	620
Whole-wheat bread crumbs, ½ cup	22	70
Chopped broccoli, 2 cups	288	80
Beaten whole egg, 1	27	82
Dash of pepper	—	—
Lemon juice, 2 tbsps.	—	—
Parmesan cheese, 2 tbsps.	138	46
Four servings:	1337	898
One serving:	334	225

Drain and flake salmon; put into large bowl. Add remaining ingredients, except cheese. Grease a 9″ × 5″ × 3″ loaf pan. Pour mixture into pan. Top with cheese. Bake at 350° for 30 minutes.

SARDINE SALAD

	Calcium, in mg.	Calories
Sardines, 4 oz.	496	232
Mash with		
Minced onion, 1 tsp.	8	7
Dijon mustard, ½ tsp.	—	—
Lemon juice, 1 tbsp.	1	5
Pepper, ¼ tsp.	5	2
One serving:	510	246

SPINACH SQUARES

	Calcium, in mg.	Calories
Fresh spinach, 1 lb.	422	100
Low-fat cottage cheese, 1 cup	138	165
Low-fat yogurt, ½ cup	150	75
Grated low-fat Cheddar cheese, 2 oz.	422	160
Beaten egg whites, 2	6	34
White wine, 1 oz.	—	13
Wheat germ, 1 tbsp.	—	13

Spinach Squares *(con't)*

	Calcium, in mg.	Calories
Dijon mustard, 1 tsp.	—	—
Black pepper, ½ tsp.	9	5
Grated Parmesan cheese, 3 tbsps.	207	69
Paprika	—	—
Eight servings:	1354	651
One serving:	169	82

Tear spinach into small pieces. Combine yogurt, cheese, wine. Mix spinach with cheese. Add pepper and mustard. Pour into square 8-inch baking dish. Top with wheat germ, grated cheese and paprika. Bake at 350° for 30 minutes. Serves eight.

Stuffed Tomato

	Calcium, in mg.	Calories
Tomatoes, 4	80	120
Skim-milk ricotta, ½ cup	335	170
Low-fat Mozzarella, 2 oz.	417	160
Pamesan cheese, 1 oz.	320	110
Tofu, 4 oz.	144	90
Brown rice, ½ cup	9	90
Lemon juice, 2 tbsps.	—	10
V-8 juice, 2 oz.	7.5	20
Pepper, ¼ tsp.	—	—
Oregano, 1 tsp.	30	4
Basil, 1 tsp.	24	5
Four servings:	1222	779
One serving:	305	194

Cut off tops of tomatoes, scoop out insides. Put insides into blender, add ricotta, Mozzarella, tofu, lemon juice and seasonings. Do not let mixture get puréed. Put mixture into bowl, add rice and half the Parmesan cheese. Pour 2 ounces of V-8 into the bottom of the baking dish. Stuff tomatoes with mixture. Sprinkle with basil, lemon juice and remainder of the Parmesan. Bake at 350° for 30 minutes. Serves four.

STUFFED TOMATO WITH SALMON

	Calcium, in mg.	Calories
Tomatoes, 2	40	66
Canned salmon, 1 cup	431	310
Brown rice, ½ cup	9	90
Parsley, 2 tbsps.	30	5
Yogurt, ½ cup	150	75
Grated low-fat cheese, 1 oz.	207	80
Parmesan cheese, 2 tbsps.	138	46
Minced garlic, 1 tsp.	—	—
Paprika	4	12
V-8 or tomato juice, 2 oz.		
Two servings:	1009	684
One serving:	504	342

Cut off tops of tomato, scoop out insides. In a large bowl, flake salmon, add tomato insides, yogurt, parsley, garlic and cheese; mix in the rice. Stuff everything into the tomato. Pour tomato juice or V-8 juice into the bottom of the baking dish. Add stuffed tomatoes. Top each with 1 tbsp. Parmesan cheese and paprika. Bake at 350° for 30 minutes. Serves two.

TOFU CHEESE SALAD

	Calcium, in mg.	Calories
Jarlsberg cheese, 2 oz.	544	180
Another low-fat cheese of choice, 2 oz.	420	180
Tofu, 4 oz.	150	90
Cucumber, 1	26	16
Tomato, 1	20	33
Carrot, 1	37	48
Paprika	—	—
Grated Parmesan cheese (for topping), 1 tbs.	69	25
Dressing		
Juice of 1 lemon	—	10
Juice of 1 lime	—	10
Low-fat yogurt, ½ cup	150	75

TOFU CHEESE SALAD *(con't)*

	Calcium, in mg.	Calories
Dijon mustard, 1/2 tsp.	—	—
Tarragon, 1/2 tsp.	—	—
Marjoram, 1/2 tsp.	—	—
Total for 1-cup serving:	466	216

Dice cheese and tofu into small cubes. Chop vegetables. Mix vegetables together with cheese and tofu. In a separate bowl or blender, combine dressing ingredients. Blend until smooth. Pour dressing over cheese mixture. Sprinkle with paprika and 1 tbsp. Parmesan. Chill.

TOFU DRESSING

	Calcium, in mg.	Calories
Tofu, 3 1/2 oz.	128	80
Low-fat yogurt, 1/2 cup	150	75
Grated carrot, 1/2	18	25
Dijon mustard, 1/2 tsp.	—	—
Dill, 1/2 tsp.	—	—
Juice of 1/2 lemon	—	10
One 2-oz. serving:	50	30

Blend all ingredients in blender at slow speed for 10 to 15 seconds.

VEAL PARMESAN

	Calcium, in mg.	Calories
Veal cutlets, 4 oz.	10	180
Oil, 1 tbsp.	—	125
Wheat germ, 1 tbsp.	—	33
Tomato sauce, 1/2 cup	6	50
Part-skim Mozzarella cheese, 1 oz., sliced	207	80
Total	223	468

Sauté cutlets in oil until golden brown. Place in baking dish, cover with sauce and cheese. Bake at 350° for 30 minutes.

WALNUT CHEESE LOAF

	Calcium, in mg.	Calories
Brown rice, 1 cup	18	178
Ground walnuts, 1 cup	100	650
Grated Cheddar cheese, 1 cup (2 oz.)	422	224
Lemon, 2 tbsps.	—	10
Beaten eggs, 2	54	164
Grated carrot, 1	51	48
Chopped celery, 1 stalk	25	9
Chopped apple, 1	12	90
Caraway seeds	14	7
Six servings:	696	1380
One serving:	116	230

Combine all ingredients. Mix well. Place in oiled loaf pan. Bake at 350° for 30 minutes. Serves six.

Magical ways to put calcium into your diet

1. Make sugar-free hot-chocolate mixes (i.e., Swiss Miss, Alba, Ovaltine) with skim milk instead of water.
2. Steam skim milk with cinnamon.
3. Make a shake with skim milk, yogurt and fresh fruit.
4. Have cereal and milk for breakfast.
5. Use cottage cheese, farmer cheese, or ricotta cheese as a spread instead of butter or margarine.
6. Melt cheese on crackers, rice cakes, breads and English muffins.
7. Have yogurt for a snack.
8. Mix fresh fruit into yogurt with ITP blackstrap molasses.
9. Use sesame seeds on vegetables, rice, salads.

10. Top vegetables and salads with grated Parmesan cheese (it's especially good on baked potatoes).
11. Add a slice of cheese to sandwiches.
12. Add more milk to coffee and tea.
13. Make salad dressings with yogurt, tofu or cottage cheese.
14. Add cubed tofu and/or cheese to salads.
15. Include a dark leafy vegetable in your daily menu.
16. When having a sweet dessert, use ice milk, frozen yogurt, pudding.
17. Flavor skim milk with vanilla or almond extract.

FIVE

Weight-Bearing Exercise

—

The second vital element in building peak bone mass is regular weight-bearing exercise. Astronauts in space get plenty of exercise, but still lose bone mass. Mechanical loading—weight on the bones—is an important element in any exercise program designed to prevent osteoporosis.

The evidence is still sketchy and more studies need to be done, but all the available results strongly suggest that exercise increases bone mass. Athletes, for example, generally have denser bones than nonathletes. A study involving elderly nursing-home patients found that those who participated in exercises actually added bone mass, while those who didn't lost bone. Some experts feel these data are less than totally convincing, and the results of the nursing-home study have yet to be duplicated elsewhere, but most doctors would agree that exercise *probably* aids the formation of bone mass. Past studies have conclusively demonstrated that inactivity and immobilization lead to rapid bone loss, so even if exercise turns out not to be a factor in adding bone, it's definitely a good idea to protect yourself against bone loss. It's also been suggested that exercise leads to more efficient absorption of calcium.

Any kind of weight-bearing exercise, provided you don't overdo it, will help protect your bone mass and guard against osteoporosis. If you're one of those people who's bored silly by floor work or exercise machines and prefers to bicycle to work every day or dance the night away at your local club four times a week, don't worry: you're probably giving your bones all the stress they need to keep them strong. As far as the dancing goes, however, if your idea of a night out includes four drinks as well as all that dancing, you're most likely undoing all the good the exercise is doing you.

Bicycle riding, weight lifting, aerobic dancing, rope skipping and calisthenics are all fine; swimming is less beneficial, since the water supports most of your weight. Such high-intensity activities as jogging are certainly good exercise, but the increased risk of trauma from the pounding your bones take makes them a less-than-ideal type of exercise for osteoporosis prevention.

Forms of Weight-Bearing Exercise

Aerobic dancing	Jumping rope
Bicycling	Rowing
Calisthenics	Weight training on
Canoeing	machines such as
Free-weights training	Nautilus and
Gymnastics	Universal
Hiking	Walking
Jogging	

How to Tell If You're Exercising Too Much

How much exercise should you get? As much as you like, basically; twenty minutes three times a week is normally considered the minimum for fitness. There's one very important sign to watch for that tells you you're exercising too much: any drastic change in the frequency, nature or duration of your menstrual cycle. Many women athletes have menstrual problems associated with loss of fat, and there are several studies indicating that women who are amenorrheic (not menstruating at all) and continue to exercise are depleting their bones of vital minerals, including calcium. Any woman who exercises regularly and finds that her periods are becoming irregular or are disappearing should cut down on her activity and consult her doctor. Unless this happens, however, the more exercise the better, as far as your bones are concerned. Of course, you should consult with your doctor before starting any exercise program.

Exercises That Build Stronger Bones

There are specific areas of the body that are particularly susceptible to osteoporotic fractures: the spine, site of crush fractures (those dowager's humps that make older women stoop); the wrist, another delicate spot; and the hip, location of the most serious kinds of osteoporotic fractures, the ones that have a 15–30 percent mortality rate. Specific exercises can help you strengthen the muscles that support these bones, as well as the bones themselves.

If you have been inactive, start very slowly. You can always build up the number of exercises that you do. Remember, this is a lifetime activity, not a two-week crash program. Warm up before exercising and cool down afterward. Use leg warmers.

These exercises do not constitute a complete program of physical fitness, but they concentrate on the areas of the body where osteoporotic fractures most commonly occur. Since the exercises are reasonably vigorous, you should try them only if you're in good health; they're certainly *not* designed for someone who already has osteoporosis or who suspects that her bones may be fragile. That doesn't mean women in less-than-perfect health shouldn't exercise; they should try the gentler activities recommended in Chapter 8.

A calcium-rich diet and regular weight-bearing exer-
(continued on page 106)

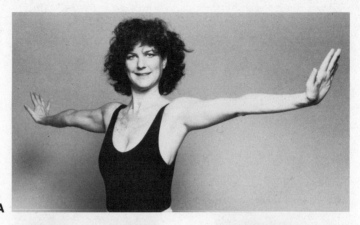

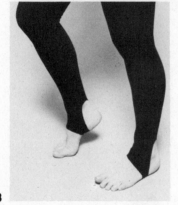
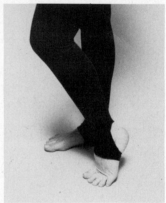

Pushing the Walls Away
For Arms and Wrists

(These arm exercises are also very good for your heart.)

1. Extend your arms to the sides at shoulder height with the hands flexed; your elbows should be straight and your hands as close to right angles with your arms as you can make them. **(Fig. A)**

2. Begin walking your feet, making sure that you rise all the way up on your toes and then go all the way down on your heels with each movement. **(Fig. B, C)**

84

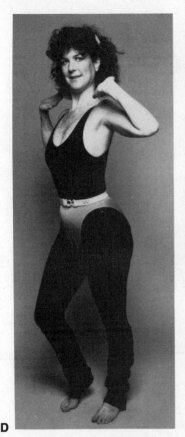
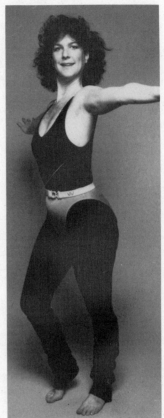

D   E

3. In time to the movement of your feet (music helps with all these exercises), bring your flexed hands in to your shoulders **(Fig. D),** then push them away toward the walls **(Fig. E).** Repeat eight times.

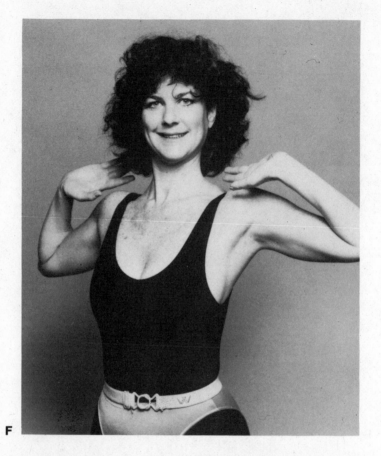

F

4. Then bring your hands to your shoulders **(Fig. F)** and push the flexed palms up toward the ceiling, straightening the arms **(Fig. G),** eight times.

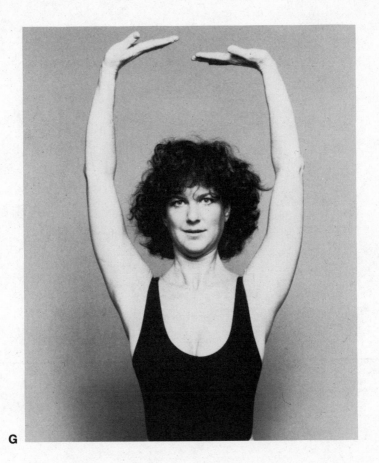

G

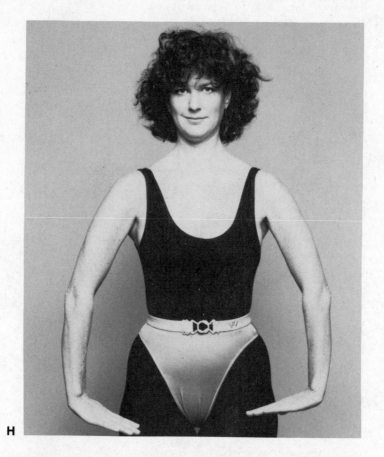

H

5. Now push your palms toward the floor **(Fig. H),** then raise them to just under your armpits **(Fig. I)** and extend again, eight times.

Repeat the entire exercise with four counts, then do the series with two repetitions of each motion, then finish with single counts—eight repetitions of the hands flexed a single time to the side, then up, then down, to complete the exercise. Remember to keep treading your feet; the blood circulates better.

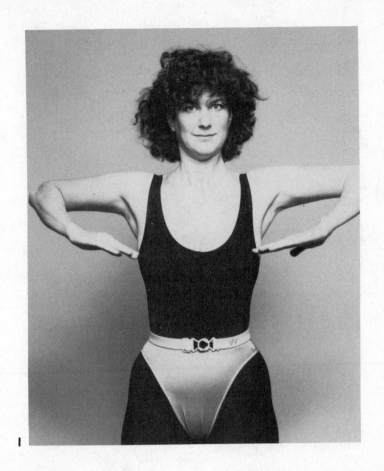

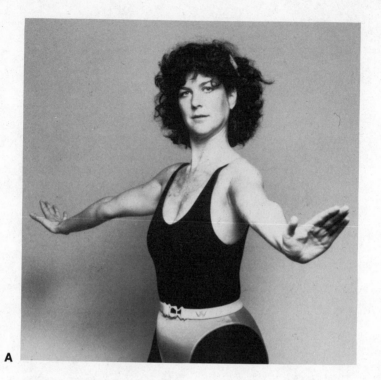

A

Arm Circles
For Arms and Wrists

1. Extend your hands to the sides at shoulder height, palms
flexed, and circle the arms forward in tight, quick movements
that keep time with the treading of your feet. **(Figs. A, B, C)**
Circle forward sixteen times, then reverse and circle back for
sixteen counts. Keep the arms straight and the feet moving as
you repeat the two circles: eight times forward and back, then
four times each, then two. (If this is too much for you, begin with
eight counts and work down from there.)

2. Now loosen up the shoulders and arms with a few big, wide
circles in either direction; you can do these more slowly.

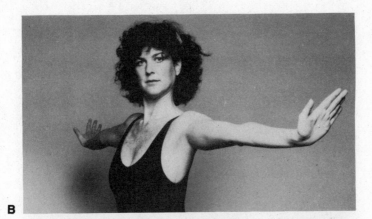

B

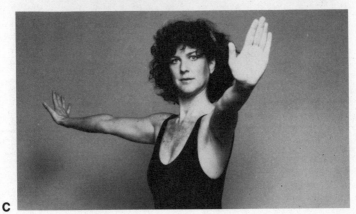

C

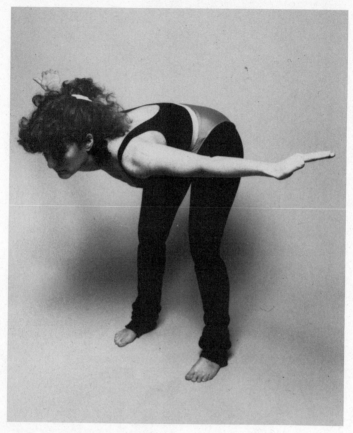

A

Back and Beyond
For the Back

1. Stand with your feet parallel to each other, about hip width apart.

2. Now bend your knees and lean over from the lower back, so that your back is in a straight line parallel to the floor.

3. Extend your arms to the sides so that they also make a straight line parallel to the floor. **(Fig. A)**

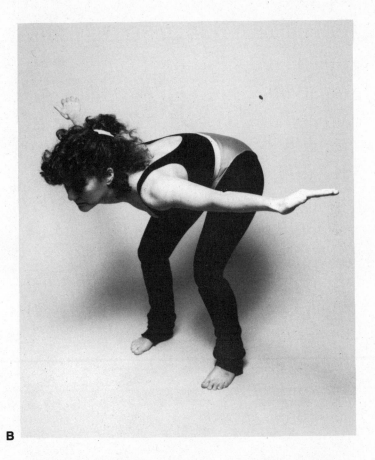

B

4. Pulse gently (*don't* bounce vigorously) on the knees for two counts; remember, your back and arms are straight at all times. **(Fig. B)**

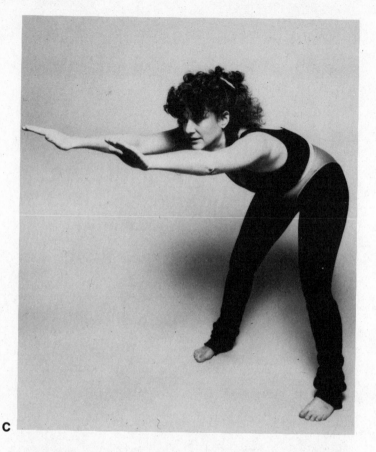

C

5. Now drop the arms and pulse them through your legs for two counts, trying to bend out of the lower back rather than hunching over to get your arms through your legs. **(Figs. C, D)**

6. Now straighten the back, extend the arms, and repeat the first pulsing movement two times; then pulse through your legs again.

Do this as many times as you can—eight or so to start—and don't be lazy, even though your thighs will hurt after a few repetitions. Don't overdo it, however; your back shouldn't hurt at all if you're extending it properly. Concentrate on keeping it straight.

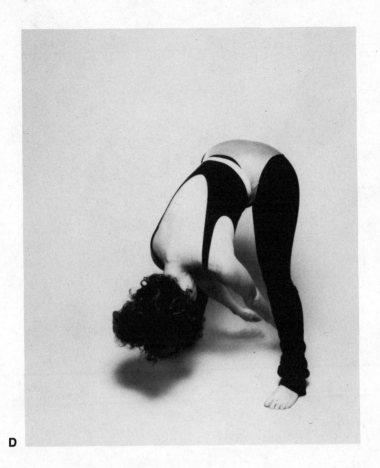

D

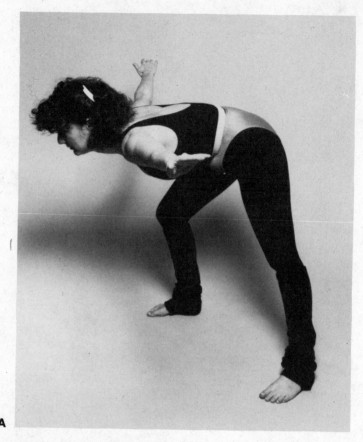

A

Side to Side
For Back, Legs and Arms

1. Stand with your legs slightly wider apart than in "Back and Beyond," still with your back extended straight in front of you and your arms straight out to either side.

2. Straighten the left knee and bend the right, shifting all the weight to your right side and keeping the back and the arms motionless. **(Fig. A)**

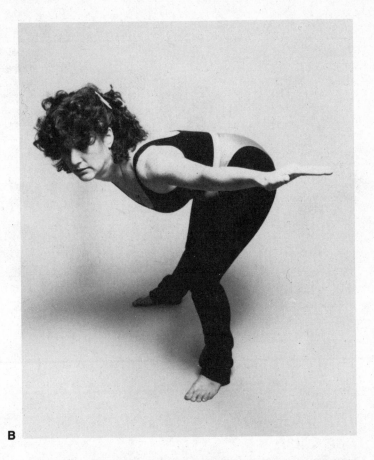

B

3. Pulse on the right knee twice, then straighten it, shift your weight and bend the left knee **(Fig. B),** pulsing twice on that side.

Repeat the sequence eight times or more. If you have a weak back, it may take you a while to be able to do Exercises 3 and 4 correctly. Concentrate on keeping the back as straight as possible; if you're subject to backaches, these exercises will be a big help.

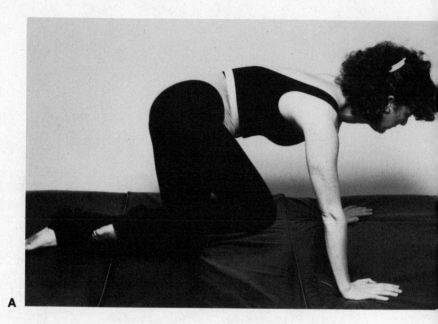

A

Leg Curls
For Back, Hips, Buttocks, Stomach and Legs

1. Get down on your hands and knees: arms shoulder width apart and straight, legs hip width apart, back straight (neither arched down nor contracted up).

2. Now draw your right knee in to your chest **(Fig. A),** then extend it in the air straight in back of you **(Fig. B).** Don't lift it any higher than is comfortable and *don't* lift your head or arch your back as you extend the leg.

Repeat this motion eight times, then repeat the series on the left side. Do eight more on each side if you can.

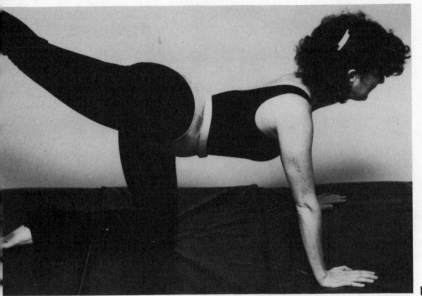

B

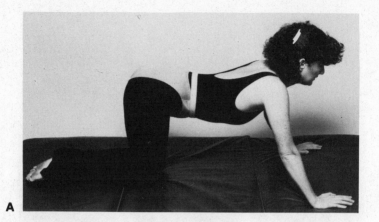

A

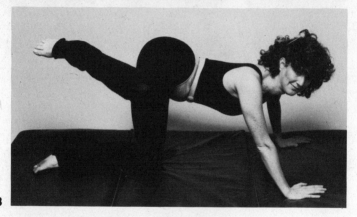

B

Side Lifts and Side Kicks
For Hips, Buttocks and Legs

1. On your hands and knees **(Fig. A),** lift your right knee up sideways to shoulder height (the leg is still bent) **(Fig. B),** then return it to starting position; repeat eight times, trying not to lean into the left hip as you lift the right leg.

2. Repeat the series on the left side—again, trying not to lean into the opposite hip as you lift the leg. Be very conscious of your back, which should be straight, not arched.

100

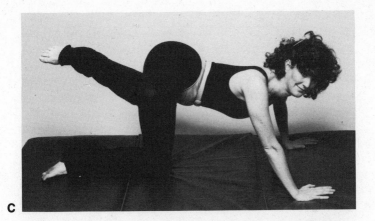

C

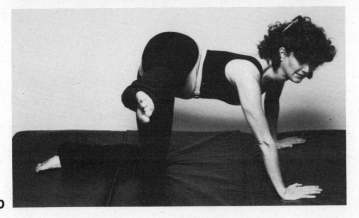

D

3. If you're feeling really strong, hold the right leg up at shoulder height, still bent **(Fig. C),** then extend the foot so the leg is now extended straight from the hip **(Fig. D).** Bend the leg in, keeping it at shoulder height, and repeat eight times. This little extension is great for the muscles around the buttock and the hip. It should never hurt your back, however; if it does, stop immediately.

101

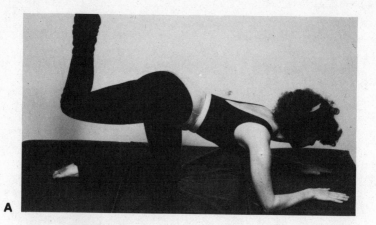

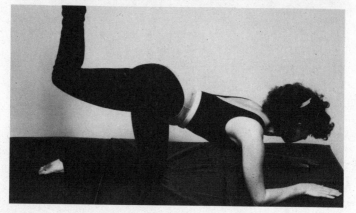

Knee Pulses
For Hips, Buttocks, Stomach and Thighs

1. On your hands and knees, lower yourself onto your elbows in front, in order not to put pressure on your lower back. Lift your bent right leg up in back of you to hip level, with the knee pointing to the floor and the toe pointing to the ceiling. **(Fig. A)**

2. Pulse the leg up, always bent, eight times; then repeat on the left side. **(Fig. B)**

Try not to let the bent leg drop below hip level at the bottom of the pulse, and make sure your knee is pointing straight down. Don't arch your back, and stop if your lower back hurts at all.

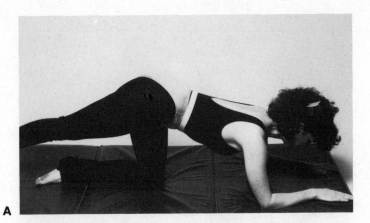

A

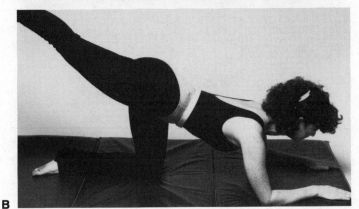

B

Leg Lifts
For Legs, Hips and Back

Stretch everything out a little in this next exercise.

1. Keep your elbows on the floor and extend your right leg straight in back of you, with the toe touching the floor. The left leg remains bent underneath you. **(Fig. A)**

2. Life the right leg up as high as it will comfortably go **(Fig. B)**, then lower it to the floor.

Repeat eight times at a reasonably brisk pace; then repeat the series on the left side.

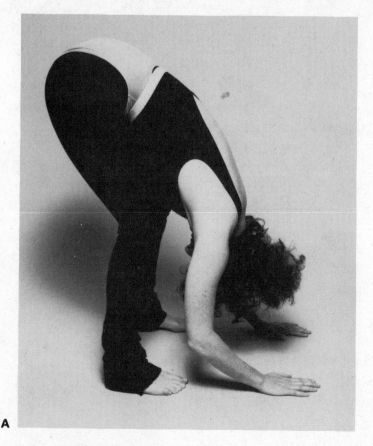

A

Stretching Out

1. Stand with your knees bent, your palms on the floor and your heels either touching the floor or as close to the floor as you can get them. **(Fig. A)**

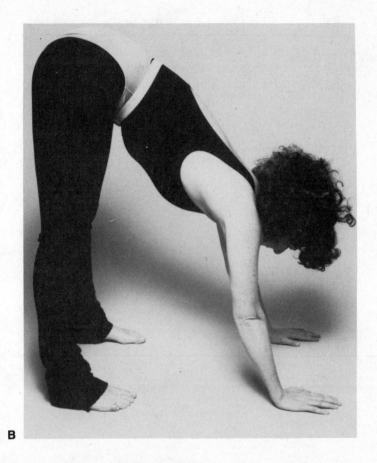

B

2. Straighten your knees, keeping your palms on the floor (or as close to it as you can), and stretch over for four counts. **(Fig. B)**

Repeat four times before you stand up and shake everything out.

cise in the essential years before age thirty-five will help you achieve your peak bone mass, the maximum amount of bone your genetic background will allow. It can't be emphasized too strongly that this is the single most important element in preventing osteoporosis. As we'll see in Chapter 8, once the damage is done to your bones there's only a limited amount that doctors can do to repair it. Building stronger, healthier bones *before* menopause is the key to osteoporosis prevention.

SIX

Preventing Bone Loss During and After Menopause

—

If the years before thirty-five are the most important in preventing osteoporosis (and you should continue to practice the good habits you developed then all through your thirties and forties), those during and after menopause are nearly as crucial. By the time you reach menopause, your peak bone mass is history—you've lost some of it already, in fact—but it's possible to avoid the accelerated postmenopausal bone loss that causes so many women to develop osteoporosis. The physical changes you go through at menopause can radically increase age-related bone loss, but proper diet, exercise and (possibly) medical treatment will protect your bone mass.

Why You Need More Calcium at Menopause
At menopause, estrogen levels fall dramatically. We've already discussed the role estrogen plays in protecting bone mass and facilitating the absorption of calcium; as its presence in the body declines, your bones lose calcium, and the mineral is no longer absorbed well from your diet. Older people don't absorb calcium efficiently in any case; the loss of estrogen in older women exacer-

bates this problem. All postmenopausal women need to keep their calcium intake up, and women who aren't getting estrogen replacement therapy (its pros and cons are examined in detail below) should actually *increase* their intake to 1500 mg. of calcium daily. In some studies, calcium has been shown to suppress age-related bone loss and lower the fracture incidence in patients with osteoporosis all by itself. In any case, at a period in your life when bone resorption is increasing and calcium absorption is decreasing, it's essential to make sure your body gets sufficient dietary calcium.

Calcium Supplements

The calcium-rich foods listed on pages 50–53 should continue to be an important part of your diet, but 1500 mg. is a lot of calcium, and at menopause you may want to consider taking calcium supplements as well. You should take only enough to bring your total calcium intake to 1500 mg.; if you get 1000 mg. in your diet, take only 500 mg. in supplemental form. This is important, because people with excessive levels of calcium in the blood are more prone to calcification in the arteries, which can lead to arteriosclerosis (hardening of the arteries), a health problem to which every older person should be alert.

There are several different types of calcium supplement; they vary primarily in the percentage of calcium they contain. Calcium carbonate tablets are 40 percent calcium, calcium lactate 13 percent, calcium gluconate only 9 percent. Doctors often prefer the carbonate variety, simply because its higher percentage means fewer pills to take and better chances for patient compliance. In terms of convenience and expense, calcium carbonate is probably the best choice for you, too, and you should be aware that several major brands of antacid (*not* the ones containing aluminum) have just as much right to be called calcium carbonate as the more expensive products marketed by the various drug companies. You may feel a little silly taking Tums, for example, as a calcium supplement, but it's a lot cheaper than many of the more fancily packaged tablets.

The one problem that some women have with calcium carbonate tablets is that at high dosages they sometimes cause constipation and/or flatulence. If that's the case, calcium gluconate, although considerably more expensive, is less constipating. Chelated-calcium tablets, which supposedly make the calcium easier to absorb, haven't been proven to do any such thing—and, unsurprisingly, they cost more. A 1982 report found lead contamination in samples of bone meal and dolomite, two other kinds of calcium supplement; they should be avoided.

You May Need More Vitamin D
In general, as you get older the delicately balanced system for calcium sufficiency described in Chapter 1 works less well. Women have particular problems because of the drop in their estrogen levels, but there are other factors as well. Calcitonin secretions, which dis-

Not Getting Enough Calcium	Getting Plenty of Calcium
Calcium in the blood drops	Calcium in the blood rises
PTH level rises—bones release calcium (resorption)	PTH level drops—no calcium is released from bones
Calcitonin levels drop—bones are not protected against resorption	Calcitonin levels rise—bones are protected against resorption
More hormonal vitamin D_3 produced, dietary calcium absorbed better into bones	Less hormonal vitamin D_3 produced, calcium absorbed less efficiently

Calcium supplements
Listed by types; within types, listed in order of increasing cost.

Product (manufacturer)	Calcium per tablet	Cost of 1000 mg.
Calcium carbonate tablets		
Tums Antacid (Norcliff-Thayer)	200 mg.	$ .12
Caltrate 600 (Lederle)	600	.18
Biocal (Miles)	500	.21
Calcium Carbonate (Lilly)	260	.23
Alka-2 Chewable Antacid (Miles)	200	.27
Os-cal (Marion)	500	.27
Biocal (Miles)	250	.34
Calcium lactate tablets		
Calcium Lactate (General Nutrition Corp.)	100	.26
Natural Calcium Lactate (Schiff)	100	.28
Formula 81 (Plus)	83	.40
Calcium Lactate (Lilly)	84	.55
Calcium gluconate tablets		
Calcium Gluconate (Pioneer)	62	.56
Calcium Gluconate (Lilly)	47	1.51
"Chelated" calcium tablets		
Chelated Calcium (Solgar)	167	.35
Calcium Orotate 2000 (Nature's Plus)	100	1.70
Calcium Orotate (Kal)	50	2.33

courage the release of calcium from the bones, decline, while parathyroid hormone (PTH) secretions, which encourage resorption, seem to rise. Most importantly, the need for vitamin D to properly absorb calcium increases with age. Postmenopausal women should make sure they're exposed for at least 15 minutes a day to sunlight, which stimulates formation of vitamin D, and they may want to increase the amount of vitamin D

togen treatment will cause regular withdrawal bleeding similar to a menstrual period, which many women find annoying. And as far as estrogen's role in preventing potentially fatal fractures is concerned, remember that hip fractures, which are the ones with high mortality rate, seldom occur with any frequency before age seventy, some twenty years after most women go through menopause.

Given women's past experiences with birth control pills (although the dosage of estrogen in postmenopausal therapy is much lower), the pros and cons of estrogen replacement therapy should be weighed very carefully indeed before proceeding with such a drastic and long-term treatment. Women who are at particularly high risk of osteoporosis, those with a family history of the disease or who have a large number of other risk factors mentioned in Chapter 2, may feel that in their case it makes sense to undergo a therapy that has been demonstrated to effectively prevent accelerated bone loss. It seems far less persuasively indicated for women whose calcium intake has been sufficient in the premenopausal years, who get plenty of exercise and who don't display many of the risk factors of osteoporosis.

*   *   *

Menopause is a difficult period for many women. Your body is going through a lot of changes, some of which can be traumatic both physically and emotionally. The increased risk of osteoporosis in these years is simply one more problem to worry about, but it's a problem you can avoid if you're careful to stick to your calcium-rich diet and continue to exercise regularly. Whether or not you wish to have estrogen replacement therapy is a decision you must make yourself: don't make it lightly.

Osteoporosis Prevention Checklist
1. Make sure you get the recommended daily amount of calcium, either in your diet or in calcium tablets. (See page 42.)
2. Do at least 20 minutes of weight-bearing exercise at least three times a week. (See pages 84–105.)
3. Get at least 15 minutes of sunshine each day, to ensure that your body is getting enough vitamin D. As you get older, consider taking a vitamin-D supplement *if* your doctor thinks you need it. (See pages 109–111.)
4. Avoid alcohol, caffeine and nicotine as much as possible. (See page 33.)
5. Don't take aluminum-containing antacids. (See page 33.)
6. Watch your diet carefully; avoid getting excess amounts of protein, phosphorus, fat and oxalic acid. (See pages 34–35.)
7. Make sure you get enough magnesium in your diet. (See page 44.)
8. Consider estrogen replacement therapy after menopause if you are in a high-risk group for osteoporosis. (See pages 111–113.)

PART III

If You Develop Osteoporosis

SEVEN

How to Know If You Have Osteoporosis

———

Despite your best preventive efforts, you may still develop osteoporosis at some point in your post-menopausal years. All the measures I've discussed will reduce the risk of osteoporosis, but of course they can't eliminate it. One expert points out that some of his patients with dangerously low bone mass have absolutely no risk factors in their background to explain their bones' depleted state; he speculates there are as-yet-undiscovered genetic factors involved in the development of osteoporosis.

Prevalance and Incidence

At first glance, the percentage of elderly women with osteoporosis is frighteningly high. A 1969 study in Michigan found that 39.2 percent of its female subjects between the ages of fifty and fifty-four showed evidence of spinal osteoporosis; 57.7 percent of those aged fifty-five to fifty-nine showed the same signs; 65.5 percent of those sixty to sixty-four; 73.5 percent ages sixty-five to sixty-nine; 84.2 percent of those between seventy and seventy-four; and an incredible 89 percent in the seventy-five-and-older age bracket. The problem is serious, but not quite as bad as those percentages suggest. For

Prevalence Rates*
of Osteoporosis in Michigan Women of Age 45 and
Older, by Age Group

Age Group (in Years)	Number of Women in Study	Percentage with Osteoporosis
45–49	290	17.9
50–54	309	39.2
55–59	514	57.7
60–64	426	65.5
65–69	299	73.5
70–74	177	84.2
75	73	89.0
Total	2,088	56.7

*Prevalence rates are based on X rays of the dorso-lumbar spine.
Source: A. P. Iskrant and R. Smith, Jr. "Osteoporosis in Women 45 Years and Over Related to Subsequent Fractures." *Public Health Report* 84:33–38, 1969.

one thing, osteoporosis is often asymptomatic; many of those women with bone mass low enough to be classified as osteoporotic will never break a bone or acquire a dowager's hump at all. Only one person in three with osteoporosis will ever progress to develop fractures or other symptoms. Still, the odds are bad enough. Approximately 1.7 percent of those between ages forty-five and sixty-four, and 2 percent aged sixty-five and older, have a fracture due to osteoporosis *each year*. In the population over age seventy-five, 1–2 percent each year will fracture a hip; 40 percent of them will die within two years of the injury. The fact that most people with low bone mass don't ever get osteoporotic fractures is small consolation to the unlucky ones who do.

How to Know If You Have Osteoporosis Before You Break a Bone

Osteoporosis is basically asymptomatic until a fracture occurs—and who wants to find out then? Medical efforts are now increasingly bent toward identifying those at greatest risk of osteoporosis while it's still early enough for them to do something to prevent it. This hasn't yet happened, but there are a few warning signals that may indicate you have osteoporosis before you break a bone. If you notice that you have any of these symptoms, you should consult a doctor immediately and arrange for more definite tests to check for osteoporosis.

The first warning signal is a constant, localized pain in your lower back, which may mean you have spinal osteoporosis. Most ordinary backaches tend to spread out as muscle fatigue increases; the backache that's symptomatic of spinal osteoporosis doesn't radiate.

The principal symptom of spinal osteoporosis is loss of height. If you're becoming stooped from the waist, it's a good bet that you've had crush fractures in your spine without realizing it. (These vertebral fractures are sometimes—alas, not always—painless, so you don't know you've had them.) If you measure yourself and find you're an inch shorter than you remembered, it's time to make an appointment with your doctor to check for osteoporosis.

Since your teeth are made of bone, as is your jaw, sometimes osteoporosis can cause periodontal problems. The jaw isn't the most common site for osteoporosis, and plenty of people who have periodontal difficulties don't have osteoporosis, so don't jump to conclusions. A postmenopausal woman who's never had dental trouble and suddenly finds she has loose teeth, however, should check with her doctor. It just might be an early symptom of osteoporosis.

Again, if you notice any of these symptoms, consult your doctor immediately for further testing.

Have Your Bone Density Measured
The next step to take if you suspect you may have osteoporosis is to undergo some form of bone density measurement. There are many ways to do this, but two relatively recent techniques currently seem best: com-

puterized axial tomography (also known as a CAT scan) and dual photon absorptiometry. Neither method measures bone density directly; they gauge the bone's mineral content, which is linked to the bone mass in a constant relationship. In osteoporosis, unlike some other bone diseases, the amount of mineral in a given amount of bone remains the same; when the mineral content is low, it means there isn't as much bone as there used to be. If your bone mineral content—and hence your bone mass—is found to be below a certain level, you have osteoporosis.

"The ideal technique for monitoring bone mass non-invasively [i.e., without taking out a piece of bone] in osteoporosis is one that quantitates primarily trabecular bone at [the] spine and possibly hip," writes one authority considering the advantages of various methods. By this standard, CAT scanning is particularly good. It measures the inner portion of the spinal vertebrae, which is primarily trabecular bone; dual photon absorptiometry by contrast measures the entire vertebrae, including cortical bone and possibly some of the surrounding tissue. The CAT scan equipment is available in more hospitals than dual photon, so it's easier to find. It's not cheaper, however: a single-energy CAT scan costs $150–175, while dual photon absorptiometry is slightly lower at $125. (None of the methods for measuring bone mass is inexpensive.)

The accuracy of a single-energy CAT scan is less than perfect. Dual-energy CAT scanning is more accurate, but both types have relatively high doses of radiation: 250 millirems for single-energy, 500 for dual-energy CAT scans. Dual photon absorptiometry has a much lower dose of radiation (10 millirems) and is considered to have better accuracy. In sites where it's important to measure cortical as well as trabecular bone, like the hip, dual photon may be the best method, while CAT scanning may be preferable in the spine, where it zeroes in on the relevant area better.

Problems with Bone Density Measurements

As bone density measurements are used more often, a few problems with them have become apparent. Most importantly, no technique can predict with certainty whether or not a person will develop osteoporosis. As these measuring techniques are used more frequently, doctors should begin to get a better sense of what the normal range of bone mineral content is and what level indicates substantial risk of osteoporosis. Right now, they're unsure. They can tell you if you *have* osteoposis, but not whether you're in danger of developing it. Still, the fact that you can find out you have osteoporosis *before* you break a bone is a major step in the right direction.

Another problem is that experts have come to believe that measuring bone mass at one site may not necessarily predict bone mass at another site. Until recently, it had been assumed that bone mass was relatively uniform throughout the skeleton, which isn't the case at all. Chapter 1 included statistics on the varying rates of bone loss from the different kinds of bone; clearly, an area like the lumbar vertebrae of the spine that's losing 8 percent of its mass yearly will not have the same density as a leg bone that's losing a mere 1 percent per year. Since osteoporosis is now commonly divided into two categories, which may have different responses to treatment as well as varying rates of decline in bone mass, it becomes likely that many patients will need to have bone density measurements taken in more than one location. This, of course will increase the cost—perhaps as high as $400 in some cases.

Postmenopausal and Senile Osteoporosis

Bone density measurements are now being used not just to diagnose osteoporosis but also to evaluate the bones' responsiveness to treatment. This is one of the tools that is allowing experts to divide osteoporosis into two separate categories with increasing assurance, as they find varying responses to therapy in the two different tyes of the disease. Type I osteoporosis, in which the loss of trabecular bone is greater than that of cortical, causes spinal crush fractures and broken wrists and primarily affects women between fifty-five and seventy-five. It seems to be less responsive to calcium than to estrogen, and in fact most authorities suspect that estrogen deficiency (rather than lack of calcium) is the principal factor in the development of this kind of osteoporosis. For that reason, it's often called postmenopausal osteoporosis.

Type II osteoporosis is also referred to as senile osteoporosis, because its victims are much older (seventy to eighty-five), and it has a significant number of male sufferers, although women are still afflicted in much greater numbers. This is the kind of osteoporosis that causes hip fracture, and insufficient dietary calcium is believed to be a major factor. Impairment of the kidneys' production of the hormonal form of vitamin D_3 has also been observed; Chapter 1 showed how this active form of vitamin D increases the efficiency of calcium absorption.

Over a ten-year period, 95 percent of those postmenopausal osteoporotics who have had a spinal crush fracture will have additional fractures—as many as six in some cases. Some 75 percent of them will lose up to four inches in height. The incidence of hip fractures produced by senile osteoporosis increases steadily with age, and those breaks have a high mortality rate. They often permanently disable many of those who don't actually die from them. When the symptoms of osteoporosis finally manifest themselves, in the form of broken bones, they are severe.

EIGHT

How to Treat Osteoporosis

Osteoporosis has no cure—only treatment. Nothing currently available will give you back the bone mass that's been lost to osteoporosis, but there are several therapies the will reduce the rate of bone loss, perhaps even halt it. Most of them are familiar as preventive measures from Part II: calcium, estrogen and exercise. In addition, calcitonin, the hormone that suppresses bone resorption, was recently approved for clinical use by the Food and Drug Administration. These four therapies are your basic weapons against osteoporosis once it has developed.

Calcium Supplementation
Virtually all forms of osteoporosis treatment take calcium as their starting point. No matter what else an osteoporotic patient is given, her doctor will want to ensure that she's getting an adequate amount of calcium, either in her normal diet or through dietary supplements of calcium tablets. Calcium therapy alone has been shown in one study to halve the osteoporosis fracture rate. Calcium supplementation, therefore, is the first and most obvious step to take in the treatment

of the disease; everything else comes later. Supplements of vitamin D may also be suggested, to ensure proper calcium absorption; treatment with the hormonal form of vitamin D_3 is an experimental therapy and will be discussed in detail below.

Estrogen Replacement Therapy

The benefits and dangers of estrogen replacement therapy have been examined in Chapter 6. For women with established osteoporosis, estrogen's unquestionable effectiveness in preventing further bone loss is attractive. Since spinal osteoporosis, which is particularly common, may not be especially calcium-sensitive (this point has not been definitively decided), estrogen therapy should be considered with particularly care by women with crush fractures or low spinal bone mineral levels. They should remember that anyone undergoing estrogen replacement therapy must be very carefully monitored for signs of endometrial cancer and should have an endometrial biopsy every one or two years. If you decide estrogen makes sense for you, be careful to ask your doctor about the dosage you're getting. All evidence indicates that low doses—as low as .3 mg. per day, some authorities claim, although the standard dose is 0.625 mg.—are more than adequate to halt bone loss. Higher doses, as oral-contraceptive users have discovered, are associated with complications.

Exercise

People with established osteoporosis shouldn't be jogging or lifting weights, but moderate exercise is very good for them. Exercise has been shown to slow down the rate of bone loss and even stimulate bone formation in elderly patients. Some doctors dispute this study, but the general attitude toward exercise, even among the skeptical, is, "It may do some good, it can certainly do no harm." Walking for twenty minutes three times a week, arm crossing, sideward bends, exercises to strengthen the lower back and abdominal muscles are all appropriate forms of exercise for an osteoporotic patient. Check with your doctor on what would be best for you.

Recommended Exercises for Older Women

Brisk walking	Ping-Pong
Stationary bicycling	Rowing (on machines)
Calisthenics	Square dancing
Jogging on a	Swimming
trampoline	Water calisthenics

Rest

In addition to exercise, proper rest is very important for relief from the pain of osteoporosis. The curvature of the spine resulting from Type I (postmenopausal) osteoporosis in particular leads to back strain that can be partially alleviated by periods of horizontal rest. Try to manage without a pillow under your head; it will do more good under your knees to relieve strain on the back. Your bed should have a firm mattress too; proper support is all-important. To a certain extent, postmenopausal osteoporosis is self-limiting; the pain from the fractures and the strain they impose on the muscles will go away eventually, although the hump won't. Hip fractures, of course, are much more serious, and for people with Type II (senile) osteoporosis, bed rest all too often turns into permanent immobilization.

Developing New Therapies: Experimental Treatments

Although none of the treatments currently in use can do more than simply prevent further bone loss, there are a number of therapies in the experimental stage that may actually increase bone mass. None has yet been approved for clinical use, but studies of their effects on osteoporotic patients are under way.

Parathyroid Harmone

One experimental treatment consists of low doses of a

synthetic fragment of the parathyroid hormone. Chapter 1 showed that increased PTH secretions stimulate bone resorption, which might seem to make this an unlikely form of therapy. However, bone resorption and formation are so closely linked in the bone remodeling cycle that PTH will eventually increase bone formation through its effect on resorption, and it may even affect formation directly in ways that aren't yet known. High doses of PTH fragment (750 units a day) have been found to simply increase bone turnover in general, but lower amounts (400 units) seem to actually stimulate bone formation and increase the volume of trabecular bone, in particular.

Oral Phosphate

A related therapy, the administration of oral phosphate, increases bone turnover by stimulating PTH secretion. When combined with calcitonin, which inhibits resorption, this treatment has also been shown to increase bone formation and trabecular bone volume.

ADFR

An as-yet-untested theory of osteoporosis treatment is called "the ADFR regimen." It involves pulsing various agents into the body that will first activate (A) bone remodeling, then depress (D) the resorption phase, then leave a free (F) period for uninhibited bone formation, then repeat (R) the entire cycle. This rather theoretical treatment hasn't yet been evaluated experimentally.

Hormonal Vitamin D_3

The three treatments described above are still in the very early stages of development. Currently in a more advanced state of investigation is a treatment involving the active, hormonal form of vitamin D_3. There is evidence that many osteoporotic patients, particularly those with senile osteoporosis, aren't properly metabolizing vitamin D into its active form and therefore aren't absorbing calcium as well as they should be. At the very least, treatment with calcitriol (the generic name for this

Postmenopausal (Type I) and Senile (Type II) Osteoporosis Compared

Factors	Type of Osteoporosis	
	I	II
Age	55–75	70–85
Sex (F:M)	6:1	2:1
Type of bone loss	Trabecular > cortical	Trabecular = cortical
Main fracture types	Vertebral Wrist	Hip and other long bones Vertebral
Main cause	Estrogen deficiency	Aging
Importance of diet calcium	Low	High
Calcium absorption	Decreased	Decreased
Parathyroid function	Decreased	Increased
Abnormal vitamin-D metabolism	Secondary	Primary

active hormonal form) should improve calcium absorption, but the theory being tested in current clinical trials is that the hormone may stimulate bone formation as well. Until the study is completed and the results are submitted for FDA approval, probably in mid-1985, this remains an experimental therapy.

PEMF

Another experimental treatment, although not currently in widespread use, is called Pulsed Electromagnetic Fields, or PEMF. A specially fitted electrical device is placed over the broken bone; the pulsed field it produces is believed to help bones heal more rapidly. Although approved by the FDA in 1979, PEMF is still a highly experimental treatment, and many osteoporosis

experts consider it a questionable therapy whose benefits have yet to be conclusively established.

Sodium Fluoride

One treatment for osteoporosis that has undergone
some very extensive clinical investigation is the administration of sodium fluoride. There are several long-term
studies of this treatment, which has been fairly conclusively demonstrated to increase bone formation, especially when combined with 1000–1500 mg. of calcium
daily. It's a promising therapy, but there are some
difficulties with it. First of all, fluoride is a toxic drug,
and some 50 percent of those taking it feel significant
side effects. About 20 percent experience gastric irrita-
tion, usually just burning sensations and nausea, but
occasionally symptoms as severe as intractable vomiting
or ulcers. Even more disturbing is the fact that 30
percent of those taking fluoride get pains in their legs,
ankles or feet. This pain may be due to the intense bone
remodeling encouraged by fluoride (remember the
"growing pains" of childhood), but there are more
serious possibilities. About half of those with pain in the
lower extremities were discovered to have stress fractures; the fractures heal, but they raise the possibility
that fluoride may increase the density of trabecular bone
found primarily in the spine at the expense of cortical
bone found in the hips and the legs. Since hip fractures
are by far the most dangerous type of osteoporotic
damage, a treatment that increases their fragility, even if
it does wonders for the spine, is less than ideal. Experiments are also still investigating the possibility that the
new bone created by fluoride isn't as strong as normal
bone.

Fluoride therapy is a promising area, but there are
still many questions that need to be answered. One of
the principal clinicians involved in the investigation of
fluoride estimates that it will be another two to four
years before the drug can even be considered for FDA
approval.

*   *   *

"The first and most important message that has to get across to women is that they should stop *worrying* so much about osteoporosis," said one doctor interviewed for this book. "It's not such a terrible disease." It's easy to dismiss this comment, as one female interviewee did, as male insensitivity to a woman's-health issue, but in fact his point is well taken. No one wants to get osteoporosis: its symptoms are unpleasant and can be very serious. However, it's *not* necessarily a crippling disease.

The treatments discussed above will slow the rate of bone loss; with proper diet and exercise, osteoporosis victims can lead a relatively normal life. They don't need to be paralyzed by the fear of falling or immobilized by multiple fractures. In the future, treatments that are now experimental may be proven to restore lost bone and be approved for clinical use. Then, when a real cure exists for osteoporosis, we can truly say, "It's not such a terrible disease."

Glossary

ADFR Regimen. An experimental treatment for osteoporosis that uses various agents to affect the bone-remodeling process so that more bone will be formed. It has not yet been tested.

Alactasia. Also known as milk allergy, this condition means that the people who have it can't digest lactose, the milk sugar found in many dairy products. Since they're unable to eat one of the best food sources of calcium, people with alactasia are at higher risk for osteoporosis.

Amenorrhea. When normal premenopausal women stop having their menstrual period, they are amenorrheic. This condition usually means the body's estrogen levels have dropped drastically, and it may lead to osteoporosis, since lack of estrogen means the bones aren't protected as well against loss.

Bone Density Measurement. Since osteoporosis is a disease in which the bones become porous (not dense), bone density measurement is an important tool in finding out whether or not someone has osteoporosis. There are many different techniques for measuring bone density (see Chapter 7), but all of them involve scanning the bone to see whether it's as thick as normal bone or shows signs of the increasing porousness that can lead to osteoporosis.

Bone Mass. Bone mass equals bone density times the size of the skeleton; it's the total amount of bone you have in your body. (See Peak Bone Mass.)

BONE MEAL. A form of calcium supplement, samples of which were found to contain lead in 1982. Not recommended. (See Dolomite.)

BONE MINERAL CONTENT. What is actually measured in a bone density measurement, since the amount of mineral in the bone is directly linked to bone density.

CALCITONIN. The peptide hormone that protects bone against losing calcium through resorption. When calcium levels in the blood are high, so are calcitonin levels, so that the bones don't release more calcium into the blood. When calcium levels are low, so are calcitonin levels, so that the bones are free to release calcium, which is needed.

CALCITRIOL. A generic name for the active, hormonal form of vitamin D_3. (See Vitamin D.)

CALCIUM. The mineral—99 percent of which is found in the skeleton—that is essential to the proper development of bone. The lack of calcium is a primary factor in osteoporosis.

CALCIUM CARBONATE, GLUCONATE and LACTATE. Three different forms of calcium tablet. The main difference between them is the percentage of calcium they contain: carbonate is 40 percent calcium; lactate 13 percent; gluconate 9 percent.

CAT SCAN. The common name for computerized axial tomography, one technique for measuring bone density.

CHELATED CALCIUM. Another type of calcium supplement, which is claimed to be easier to digest but in fact seems only to be overpriced. Not recommended.

CORTICAL, or COMPACT, BONE. The external envelope of all bones, thinner and smoother than the interior. This type of bone makes up about 80 percent of the skeleton.

CORTICOSTEROIDS. Drugs commonly given to arthritis victims; they may lead to accelerated bone loss and osteoporosis.

CRUSH FRACTURE. The most common symptom of osteoporosis: the vertebrae in the spine are unable to support their weight and collapse together, forming the unsightly and often painful stoop called "dowager's hump."

DOLOMITE. Another form of calcium supplement, samples of which were also found to contain lead in 1982 (see Bone Meal). Not recommended.

DUAL PHOTON ABSORPTIOMETRY. One of the techniques for measuring bone density. (See CAT Scan.)

ENDOMETRIAL BIOPSY. A test for endometrial cancer.

ENDOMETRIAL CANCER. A cancer of the lining of the uterus; women undergoing estrogen replacement therapy are at increased risk for this cancer.

ESTROGEN. The female hormone produced by the ovaries that protects the skeleton against bone loss. The level of estrogen in the body drops dramatically at menopause.

ESTROGEN REPLACEMENT THERAPY. A low daily dosage of estrogen given to women after menopause to keep their estrogen levels up. It's controversial because of its link to endometrial cancer.

FORMATION. The process by which the bones take minerals from the blood and build up new bone tissue. (See Osteoblasts.)

HYPERPLASIA. An abnormal state of the lining of the uterus that indicates that endometrial cancer may be developing.

KIDNEY STONES. Blockage of the urinary track that can be caused by excess calcium intake.

LACTASE. The enzyme that helps people digest the milk sugar in dairy products. People without this enzyme have alactasia, or milk allergy.

LACTOSE. Another name for the milk sugar that people with alactasia can't digest.

MAGNESIUM. A mineral that, like calcium, is stored in the bones. The lack of magnesium has been suggested as a risk factor for osteoporosis.

MENOPAUSE. The transitional era in a woman's life, usually in her forties, when she ceases menstruating. The drop in estrogen production at menopause is one factor in the rapid bone loss that leads to osteoporosis.

MILK ALLERGY. See Alactasia.

ORAL PHOSPHATE. An experimental treatment for osteoporosis that seems to increase the turnover of bone, hence leading to the manufacture of more new bone.

OSTEOBLASTS. The cells in the bone that refill cavities, aiding new bone formation.

OSTEOCLASTS. The bone cells that drill pits on the surface of the bone and remove some of it.

OXALIC ACID. A substance found in such leafy vegetables as parsley, spinach and beet greens that may impair calcium absorption.

PARATHYROID HORMONE. Commonly referred to by its abbreviation PTH, the parathyroid hormone stimulates the release of calcium into the bloodstream when calcium levels are low; when calcium levels are high, PTH levels are lowered, so that the bones don't release calcium.

PEAK BONE MASS. The skeleton's achievement of its maximum size—usually reached at about age thirty-five. The greater a person's peak bone mass is, the better their chances of avoiding osteoporosis are: the more bone you have at your peak, the more you can afford to lose before developing osteoporosis.

PERIODONTAL DISEASE. Tooth problems that may be an indication of the presence of osteoporosis.

PHOSPHORUS. A mineral that has been suggested as a risk factor for osteoporosis when it appears in the diet in large quantities.

POSTMENOPAUSAL OSTEOPOROSIS. Also called Type I osteoporosis, this form of the disease occurs most commonly in women between the ages of fifty-five and seventy-five. The most common area for fractures is the spine, and the loss of trabecular bone is much greater than the loss of cortical bone in this form of osteoporosis.

PROGESTOGEN. An agent added in estrogen replacement therapy to reduce the risk of endometrial cancer; it has been suggested that progestogen increases the risk of hypertension and cardiovascular disease.

PROTEIN. An essential dietary element, protein in too great quantities increases calcium excretion and thus is a risk factor for osteoporosis.

RECOMMENDED DIETARY ALLOWANCE. The levels considered by the United States Food and Drug Administration as the correct amount of a vitamin or mineral to be taken daily.

REMODELING. The process by which bone is constantly being built up and torn down. (See Formation and Resorption.)

RESORPTION. The process by which the bones remove minerals from the skeleton and release them into the blood. (See Osteoclasts.)

RISK FACTOR. Certain physical and dietary characteristics are considered risk factors for osteoporosis because people with the disease have these characteristics more often than the general population does. A risk factor is something that increases your chances of getting osteoporosis.

SENILE OSTEOPOROSIS. Also called Type II osteoporosis, this form of the disease affects men and women over seventy. Trabecular and cortical bone are lost in equal amounts, and the most common site for fractures is the hip.

SODIUM FLUORIDE. An experimental treatment for osteoporosis that actually stimulates the creation of new bone, but has some serious side effects and has not yet been approved for clinical use.

TRABECULAR BONE. The spongy inner matrix of the bone that comprises about 20 percent of the total skeleton, trabecular bone is lost earlier and in greater amounts than cortical bone and is the most common type of bone lost in osteoporosis.

TYPE I OSTEOPOROSIS. See Postmenopausal Osteoporosis.

TYPE II OSTEOPOROSIS. See Senile Osteoporosis.

Vertebrae. The bony sections that make up the spine, and the most common sites for osteoporosis-related fractures. (See Crush Fracture.)

Vitamin D. When transformed by the liver and the kidneys into its metabolically active form—$1,25(OH)_2D_3$, or, more simply, the hormonal form of vitamin D_3—this vitamin plays an essential role in the absorption of calcium. In particular, when calcium intake from the diet is low, hormonal vitamin D_3 increases the efficiency of calcium absorption so that the body gets maximum benefit from the little calcium it's getting.

Weight-Bearing Exercise. Physical activity in which weight is placed on the bones during exercise—either by actual weight lifting, or any upright exercise where the bones support the body's weight—in order to put stress on the skeleton and encourage the formation of new bone.

A Note on Sources

Since this book is for the general reader, I haven't footnoted the material, which is technical enough without intimidating people further. I've drawn heavily on abstracts of the papers presented at the National Institutes of Health Consensus Development Conference in April 1984 and on the summarizing statement made by the conference's Consensus Development Panel. In addition, interviews with the following doctors were most helpful: Louis V. Avioli, Jewish Hospital of St. Louis and Washington University, St. Louis; Bruce Ettinger, Kaiser-Permanente Medical Center, San Francisco; Robert P. Heaney, Creighton University; Michael Kleerekoper, Henry Ford Hospital; and B. Lawrence Riggs, Mayo Clinic and Medical School.

Several books on osteoporosis and related subjects were also useful. *The Osteoporotic Syndrome: Detection, Prevention, and Treatment*, edited by Dr. Avioli (New York: Grune & Stratton, 1983), contained much of the most up-to-date information, although its medical terminology makes it a little abstruse for the lay reader. *Osteoporosis: What It Is, How to Prevent It, How to Stop It*, by Betty and Si Kamen (New York: Pinnacle Books, 1984), is heavily oriented toward health-food-style nutrition, and it draws some conclusions that don't appear to be fully warranted by the evidence, but the Kamens' knowledge is wide-ranging and impressive. *Menopause*, by Winnifred Berg Cutler, Celso-Ramon Garcia and David A. Edwards (New York: W. W. Norton, 1983), provided a useful summary of the pros and cons of estrogen replacement therapy, although the authors are far more enthusiastic about it than I am. *Pickles and Ice Cream: The Complete Guide to Nutrition During Pregnancy,* by Mary Abbott Hess and Anne Elise Hunt (New York: Dell, 1982), was helpful on the special needs of pregnant and nursing women. *Consumer Reports,* October 1984, contained a cogent account of the various calcium supplements' pluses and minuses. *Food Values of Portions Commonly Used,* by C. F. and H. N. Church (Philadelphia: J. B. Lippincott, 1975), and *Nutrition Almanac,* second edition (New York: McGraw-Hill Book Co., 1974), were the sources of the nutritional information in Chapter 3, and Randi Aaron, M.A., provided the recipes in Chapter 4.

Finally, I must particularly thank Dr. Stanton Cohn, who provided me with the NIH report and answered the questions of a layperson struggling with medical vocabulary during the writing of this book. He also read the final manuscript for factual errors. Naturally, any mistakes that remain are my responsibility, not his.

Index